Are You Ready?

ALSO AVAILABLE BY RIK ISENSEE
FROM ALYSON BOOKS

Love Between Men: Enhancing Intimacy and
Keeping Your Relationship Alive

Reclaiming Your Life: The Gay Man's Guide to Love,
Self-Acceptance, and Trust

Are You Ready?

The Gay Man's Guide to Thriving at Midlife

Rik Isensee

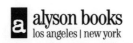

alyson books
los angeles | new york

NOTICE TO READERS

THIS BOOK IS INTENDED AS A REFERENCE VOLUME ONLY. IT IS NOT A MEDICAL MAN-
UAL. ANY HEALTH INFORMATION CONTAINED IN THIS MANUAL WAS WRITTEN TO
HELP READERS MAKE INFORMED DECISIONS ABOUT HEALTH ISSUES ASSOCIATED
WITH SEXUALITY. IT WAS NOT DESIGNED AS A SUBSTITUTE FOR ANY TREATMENT
THAT MAY HAVE BEEN PRESCRIBED BY YOUR PERSONAL PHYSICIAN. IF YOU SUSPECT
THAT YOU HAVE A MEDICAL PROBLEM, SEE A COMPETENT PHYSICIAN TO DISCUSS
YOUR CONCERNS.

© 1999 BY RIK ISENSEE. ALL RIGHTS RESERVED.

MANUFACTURED IN THE UNITED STATES OF AMERICA.

THIS TRADE PAPERBACK ORIGINAL IS PUBLISHED BY
ALYSON PUBLICATIONS INC.,
P.O. BOX 4371, LOS ANGELES, CALIFORNIA 90078-4371.
DISTRIBUTION IN THE UNITED KINGDOM BY
TURNAROUND PUBLISHER SERVICES LTD.,
UNIT 3 OLYMPIA TRADING ESTATE, COBURG ROAD, WOOD GREEN,
LONDON N22 6TZ ENGLAND.

FIRST EDITION: APRIL 1999

99 00 01 02 03 ▣ 10 9 8 7 6 5 4 3 2

ISBN 1-55583-459-0

LIBRARY OF CONGRESS CATALOGING-IN-PUBLICATION DATA
ISENSEE, RIK.
    ARE YOU READY? : THE GAY MAN'S GUIDE TO THRIVING AT MIDLIFE /
RIK ISENSEE.
    ISBN 1-55583-459-0
    1. MIDDLE AGED GAYS—UNITED STATES. I. TITLE.
HQ76.2.U5I829 1999
205.244—DC21   98-50303 CIP

COVER PHOTOGRAPH BY GIOVANNI.

CONTENTS

ACKNOWLEDGMENTS

A number of people have contributed greatly to this project. My colleagues Allan Chinen, MD, Gordon Murray, MFCC, and Paul Zak, LCSW, have all led workshops with me for gay men at midlife. During our planning and work together, we had long discussions about our own midlife issues. They kindly reviewed an earlier draft of the manuscript and gave me many valuable suggestions. I'm also grateful for feedback from other colleagues: John A. Martin, Ph.D.; Alan Sable, Ph.D.; and Diana Gray, Ph.D., who showed me her dissertation on issues confronting older lesbians. Other colleagues and friends who provided helpful insights include Michael Ahern, MFCC, Michael D'Arata, Scott Eaton, MFCC, Abraham Kanamu, Kurt Wagner, Jesse Warr, and Noe Zavala. Robert M. Kertzner, MD, is conducting research on gay men at midlife through the HIV Center for Clinical and Behavioral Studies at Columbia University. He generously provided me with some very helpful resources, including copies of his own papers, in addition to insights from his current study. My agent, Mitch Douglas at ICM, supported this idea from the beginning. Richard Labonté at A Different Light bookstore also encouraged me to pursue this project, since many gay men were asking for a book on midlife. David Groff, an editor based in New York, offered suggestions to strengthen my initial proposal and recommended it to my publisher. I would like to thank the men in my support group, who have shared their wisdom throughout our midlife process of discovery, and the many clients who inspired me with their courage in struggling with midlife challenges. And finally, I owe a great deal to the men who graciously consented to be interviewed for this project. They gave so much of their time to convey their experience and insights for the benefit of other gay men who are in the midst of this transition.

INTRODUCTION

As generations of openly gay men reach our 40s and 50s, many of us find ourselves at sea. We are no longer young, but not yet old, and it takes a while to discover who we are during this new phase of life. For men who have already been out for half their lives, it can feel odd and disorienting to be questioning their identity again. Yet it's understandable that we'd feel some trepidation, since we don't have many positive models for what it means to be gay and proud at midlife.

As a consequence, gay men may approach midlife with a sense of foreboding—a combination of embarrassment, guilt, and even shame, often reinforced by our own peers. Bombarded with images idealizing youth from both gay and mainstream media, it's easy at midlife to internalize a sense of personal failure—being over the hill, a has-been. Time to put away those disco pumps and plop on the couch, eat chocolates, and watch reruns of *I Love Lucy*.

Yet at 40 and beyond, many men arrive at a new sense of self-confidence. Gay men who have made it through this identity crisis are not as vulnerable to self-judgment or the opinions of younger men. We have wisdom from decades of experience to offer the rest of the gay community—and not just as a wise old auntie. We also have plenty to offer another man as a partner—whether just for the night or for the rest of our lives.

Gay men often experience their early years as outsiders. This tendency is also reflected in changes at midlife: We finally arrive at our own sense of self, no longer conforming to social expectations, but with a keen perspective on the surrounding culture. Just as coming out required us to get in touch with our true nature, midlife is another major juncture in the development of our identity as gay men. It's a time when many of us reflect seriously on our lives, asking ourselves: Where have I been? Where am I going? What are my true interests? And what do I want to do with the rest of my life?

This project was stimulated by seeing a number of gay clients in my psychotherapy practice whose midlife struggles resonated with my own. I thought, *Here are all these guys dealing with very similar issues, but in total isolation.* Because of denial about midlife in the gay community, many men don't realize we have a lot of reactions in common. After years of being out and about as openly gay men, they often assume they're the only ones experiencing self-doubt and uncertainty about this phase of life.

As a psychotherapist I often recommend support groups for people going through significant changes—so I decided to take my own advice and started a group for myself. Out of that experience, some colleagues and I planned a series of workshops for gay men at midlife. This combination of dealing with my own changes and listening to others inspired me to write this book.

In the course of this project, I conducted in-depth interviews with ten gay men, who shared their stories and insights about this transition (see the appendix for a brief description of each participant). Throughout the book, these men describe how they have reevaluated earlier goals and decisions in the light of a deeply felt longing for intimacy, meaningful work, and a sense of fulfillment. Although this group is not a random sample, its members span a range of ages and occupations; ethnic and racial groups; HIV status; and philosophical or spiritual beliefs. Some are in relationships, some are single, and some have had lovers die in recent years. Mostly urban dwellers now, they come from many parts of the country. All of these men have thought a great deal about these issues in their own right, so in addition to sharing personal experiences, they offer observations about midlife challenges confronting their friends and lovers as well.

There is much research still to be done about how gay men are affected by this phase of life. This book is not intended as a definitive study, but as a description of a few men's experience in the context of some larger themes that I've culled from the literature and seen in my practice. Its purpose is to help gay men counter oppressive stereotypes about growing older, affirm a positive midlife identity, and grapple more successfully with these changes.

As you will see, the men I interviewed offer some lively and differing points of view about this transition. They don't always agree with each other (or with me!), and many of their midlife dilemmas remain unresolved. There are no easy answers to the quest for meaning at this time of life. But their experiences cover a range of possibilities with warmth, wisdom, and humor.

My hope is that these observations will serve as a stimulus for reflecting on your own experience of midlife and will help you get in touch with themes that seem relevant to your journey. By working through the challenges we face at this juncture, we can recapture what was vital in our youthful ideals, tap into a rich storehouse of wisdom, and reenvision our future.

CHAPTER 1

THRIVING AT MIDLIFE

Midlife is a reflective time that offers many benefits and challenges. Most of us probably have more influence now than at any other time in our lives—in our careers, with our friends and families, and in the larger community. It's a time of life when we can reap the rewards of a lot of hard work and training. We have the self-confidence to pursue new interests as well as the maturity and wisdom to enjoy our accomplishments and relationships.

In this chapter we'll counter some misconceptions about aging in the gay community. Next we'll look at some of the positive aspects of midlife for gay men and show how these can contribute to our well-being during this transition.

Adjusting to midlife is certainly not all smooth sailing. The beginning of this passage can feel rough and tempestuous, tumbling us around and dumping us on the shore, totally disoriented. The idea is not to blame ourselves for feeling confused and demoralized at times but to see the tumult of this transforma-

tion as a developmental process. We'll look at midlife challenges in the following chapters, but having a glimpse of what
it's like to emerge on the other side can help us feel more confident about embarking on this journey.

◆   Countering Stereotypes   ◆

At midlife we're between youth and old age. In contrast to
cultures where older men are both respected and appreciated,
American culture tends to dismiss attributes and contributions
that can't easily be assigned an economic value. Our anxiety
about growing older in a culture that's not very accepting of
aging in general is compounded by homophobia.

Older gays have been the object of negative stereotyping both
from society at large and within the gay community. The image
of the lonely older man lusting after younger men is perpetuat-
ed by the right wing in an attempt to frighten and shame us into
abandoning our sexual orientation. Within the gay community
the stereotype of the "bitter old queen" divides generations—
older men are afraid of being seen as "chicken hawks," and
younger men are wary of being sexually objectified. This negative stereotype also reinforces the belief that gay relationships are
based solely on sexual attraction and that once our youth begins
to fade, we are unlikely to have any real or lasting relationships.[1]

Many gays do not buy into these beliefs, and we have evidence from various research studies that contradicts negative
assumptions about growing older in the gay community. Raymond Berger, in his book *Gay and Gray,* cited the following
findings from his own and a number of other studies:[2]

Gay men over 45 did not differ from younger gays in most aspects of psychological adjustment, and they had more stable self-concepts.[3] Most men over 65 reported satisfactory social and sex lives.[4] Most of the older gay men lived with a lover, roommates, or a family member.[5] Two fifths of the older men in one study currently lived with a lover.[6] Gay men were no more likely than heterosexual men to seek younger partners and in fact expressed a marked preference for socializing with age peers.[7]

Along similar lines, a recent study conducted by the Stop AIDS Project in San Francisco showed that there is considerable sexual interest between men of different age groups as well as a lot of interest between men the same age—including men in their 40s and 50s.[8]

Countering negative stereotypes can help us deal more successfully with our midlife transition. Realizing that growing older actually has benefits can enable us to feel less fearful about reaching out to others from different age groups. We can increase our depth of understanding through the wisdom and experience of our elders. We can also learn from younger gays by listening to their experience coming of age in a less repressive sexual climate.

♦ Positive Aspects ♦

One of the consequences of negative stereotyping is that younger men may feel dispirited and depressed about growing older. They may figure, What's the point in having safe sex or taking care of themselves in other ways, if their image of being middle-aged is so negative?[9] Yet it appears from the Stop AIDS study mentioned above that at least some young men, and a majority of gay men at midlife, actually have fairly positive attitudes about growing older. A large percentage of younger men said they were looking forward to it. Men in their 40s and 50s cited positive aspects such as maturity, wisdom, increased insight, being calmer, and feeling more relaxed.[10]

It helps to counter negative expectations not only through research findings but through the words of men who have made this transition and are feeling good about it. In the section that follows, I've outlined positive qualities that I've encountered in my interviews and included a number of accounts from the men themselves. (I'll introduce each man during his first comment, and for easy reference, these descriptions are also included in the appendix.)

Positive aspects of midlife:
- Perspective
- Self-acceptance
- Flexibility
- Knowing what's important
- Greater tolerance for ambiguity
- Less vulnerability to grandiosity and self-deprecation
- Wisdom and reflection
- Humor and healing

Perspective

By the time we've reached midlife, we have a greater perspective on our lives. The usual ups and downs of daily existence tend not to rattle us as much, simply because we've been through much of this before. Overall, there's a greater sense of equanimity.

We can see the vast changes that have taken place for gay people over the past 30 years, and that perspective enables us to appreciate our own contributions to this ongoing social revolution. Although we have a personal stake in this history, by midlife we usually have had enough experience to understand that gay liberation doesn't happen all at once—both personal and social progress in overcoming homophobia is incremental.

Kevin (Kevin is 41 and Irish-American. He loves music and cooking. He's a long-term survivor of HIV and has a partner of many years. They don't live together, and he prefers it that way): I've developed over the years the ability to see the big picture— things and people in their context. I have a greater appreciation for history and my minute place in it. I can take the bad with the good in stride. I have more understanding and humility at this age than I did when I was younger. Experience and reflection have led me to a point where I just think about things more complexly.

Brian (Brian is 50, from an Anglo-Scottish background. He just fathered a child. He has worked for the Peace Corps, as an alternative school teacher, and as a psychotherapist): Midlife gives us the best perspective we're ever going to get on life. It's the time of life when we know a lot, we've gained some power in the world, and we can see life from horizon to horizon. We can see and hold and appreciate our whole life in a way that we can't do at the beginning or at the end. And we still have physical energy and the strength and health to enjoy it. Midlife is a very busy time, because I've accumulated all these friends and interests and desires. I still have energy, but there's a gradual realization that there's not enough time left to do everything I want.

Randy (Randy is 50 and African-American. He worked for 17 years for a large corporation and recently took a severance package to explore, travel, and figure out what he'd like to do when he gets back): At midlife I feel that I make more informed choices about what kinds of jobs and relationships I want to be in. I feel more mature; I have a track record; I know what kind of person I am—what I'm good at and what I'm not, with fewer illusions than when I was younger. I'm much clearer about what I value. I'm also aware of limits—you can't have it all, so choose what you can have and go for it.

Self-Acceptance

By the time we reach midlife, earlier anxieties begin to fade. We have managed to survive a lot of disappointments as well as reap the benefits of decades of work and training. Even if we're still struggling with relationship issues, we've usually come out to friends and family, and experienced both disappointment and success. We generally feel much more accepting of our sexual orientation and our identity as gay men.[11]

Steve (Steve is 44 and Asian-American. He works as a medical researcher): I have the satisfaction of achievement, what I've already accomplished. I have less anxiety and fewer inhibitions. I never thought when I was young that I could speak in public without being completely anxious, but now I do that all the time. As I feel more comfortable with myself, I'm collaborating more with others. I'm also enjoying life—I don't have to always be productive. I don't feel the need to change as much or to push myself. I spend more on leisure time. I don't have to please everyone, because I don't care as much what other people think.

Kevin: I'm actually happier than I've ever been. I feel secure in my work, so my midlife is relatively worry-free. I like and trust myself. I feel much less vulnerable and anxious than I did when I was younger. By now I feel reasonably confident that I can do life. I've had enough difficult and anguishing experiences and survived them, so I don't feel as afraid of the world. I trust my feelings and perceptions, and I'm comfortable expressing them.

Tony (Tony is 43 and Sicilian-American. He had a lover of 14 years who died of AIDS four years ago. At 41 he went back to school to become a physician's assistant. He coparents his nine-year-old son with a lesbian couple): I have more of a sense of my own self-worth now than I used to. Through therapy and support groups, I've learned how to be honest with myself and accept myself. I'm better able to acknowledge my strong points, and I have a greater sense of fulfillment. This has grown by setting goals and achieving them, and by developing skills I didn't have as a younger person. Also, by having long-term nurturing relationships with my lover, my family, and my friends, I know others can love me over a long period of time, and this allows me to be less hard on myself.

Hal (Hal is 37, from a German and Irish background. He has worked as a chef and a carpenter, and he now runs a personal growth seminar): I feel more comfortable with who I am. There's a definite change in my level of confidence. My perspective is broader, and I have a greater acceptance of different kinds of people. I've been through enough process and change that I've learned that I just have to kick back and let it go.

Flexibility

At midlife we may experience changes in our flexibility. Because we have greater perspective, we're often less judgmental. Rather than becoming set in our ways, we find that self-reflection allows continued growth. As described in the following examples, we may have more "psychic" flexibility, in terms of how we relate to other people, but less physical flexibility, in terms of our need for sleep, recovery time from physical exertion (and partying!), or our desire for physical comfort.

Kevin: I'm vastly more flexible in a relationship. I used to be jealous and controlling and insecure. Now I'm not as threatened by my partner finding someone else attractive. I know the strong points and soft spots in my friends, and have learned to live with and even cherish their difficult parts. I think it's part of love to respect other people's vulnerability, and this view has only come with age.

Steve: Flexibility is a result of the crash I experienced, when all my usual structures were destroyed—my home, my health, and my usual way of working [see Chapter 2]. Now I'm more flexible with my schedule. I stay up late or go out on weekdays. I find myself letting go of certain ideals. I'm not cynical, but I feel less disappointed. I'm more understanding of public figures—of course people do dumb things, so I don't get so worked up about it. I accept people's faults more.

Antoine (Antoine is 45 and Hawaiian-Filipino. He works as an accountant and recently got involved with the same-sex marriage movement in Hawaii. His lover is 19 years older, and they've been together for 23 years): It depends. I'm more flexible about things that aren't a high priority. But if I have something that I really believe in, I can be inflexible. I won't make time for anything else. I focus more on what I want instead of being a part of someone else's plan.

Brian: I'm more understanding of diversity, more accepting, less judgmental about people's foibles. I feel less self-righteous about how others should change. I take a longer view of history and historical changes. I feel more flexible with people, but I need more regular sleep and can't stay up till 2 in the morning as easily as I used to. My daily living routine is pretty fixed, but I wonder what would happen if I had a boyfriend. I feel pretty settled in my house, for example, so if I met someone and we wanted to live together, would I be willing to move? Overall, I feel more physical rigidity, but greater psychic flexibility than when I was younger.

Andrew (Andrew is 48 and Anglo-American. He's a body worker who teaches Yoga and meditation): I feel more flexible when I can let go of stuff that's getting to me and realize it's not that important. That helps me recognize my patterns and not get caught up in them. I have a controlling personality, so I don't deal well with upheaval. I like measured change, not a big surprise—or even last-minute spontaneity, like a friend calling up and saying let's go to the beach when I've already planned out my day. I love change, variety, and spontaneity when I'm traveling. Just see what the day brings.

Knowing What's Important

In contrast to having more flexibility, many men reported also having a clearer idea of what's important to them. They're less willing to put up with chaos, lack of clarity in relationships, or uncertainty with their living situations. For many men, there's also a sense of urgency—to focus on accomplishing whatever it is that's really vital to them.

Steve: I'm more tolerant of people in some ways, but also less. I understand why they do absurd or thoughtless things, having done them myself, but I feel less tolerant in terms of putting up with unreliable behavior.

Mario (Mario is 42 and Latino. He's a dancer and choreographer who also works as a shipping clerk. His lover of ten years died three years ago): Having lived in the same place for 13 years, I know what I want in my home environment. I'm more intolerant of certain behaviors—like not paying rent, living in chaos, always having excuses but never following through on agreements. If someone's acting up—straighten up or get out.

Tony: When I was younger I was more open to exploring relationships with all different kinds of people. Now that I'm older, if they don't have certain qualities, I'm not interested. Compassion and kindness are the two big ones. If someone's prejudiced against different races, misogynistic, or anti-Semitic, I wouldn't pursue them.

Greater Tolerance for Ambiguity

The perseverance of youth benefits from single-mindedness—as young men, we're often cocky, self-righteous, and even dogmatic. There's a bold and rejuvenating aspect to in-your-face activism, but there's also the danger of denying self-serving

motives in ourselves and projecting them onto others. We can
see this tendency in the schisms that often occur in activist organizations, which usually start out with the best intentions but
sometimes self-destruct through internal bickering and self-
righteous purges.

At midlife we're more likely to acknowledge that our own
motives aren't always pure. As we grow older we realize that
what seemed so black-and-white when we were young men begins to take on shades of gray. We're not quite so judgmental toward conflicting ideas, and we develop a greater tolerance and
appreciation for moral ambiguity and pluralism.[12]

Randy: I'm better able to understand that people make other
choices—that doesn't make them worse, just different.

Steve: I'm more accepting of uncertainty. I don't have to be in
control all the time. I have more tolerance for ambiguity, in the
sense that I see both sides. I'm more capable of seeing the good
and the bad and tolerating both.

Mario: I have wonderful straight men friends who I've had
sex with for years—but why should I have to make them admit
they're gay? My partner and I used to be so militant. Why be so
militant and angry? I want to meet people, not put them off. If
they want my opinion, I have one, but I'm not going to shove it
down their throats.

Tony: I used to think that if someone loved me, they had to
love every part of me, and if they didn't, they didn't really love me.
I learned that they could have a hard time with certain aspects of
me and still love me. And I could do the same and still be there
for them. Now I recognize the ambiguity in myself, how I feel
about people in my life. Nothing is black or white. You have to
take the whole package, the things you like along with the things
you don't, because the things you like outweigh the other aspects.

Less Vulnerability to Grandiosity
and Self-Deprecation

As younger men, we feel the sky's the limit. Early success can lead to the belief that anything is possible. Of course, the flip side of being the greatest is being nothing at all! In the face of major disappointments, younger men are often more vulnerable to self-deprecation, instead of simply becoming more realistic.

At midlife we have more experience with success and disappointment. Reality teaches us that our initial inspiration has to be followed up with hard work if we are to get anywhere. By midlife we've usually seen some results, even though they are often more modest than what we had initially imagined. If we can recognize and appreciate what we actually have accomplished (rather than comparing our achievements with grandiose fantasies), we'll be less susceptible to tempestuous swings in self-judgment. Overall, we generally have more emotional resilience in the face of setbacks and disappointments.

Kevin: My life has basically been on more of an even keel than ever before. My self-esteem fluctuated so painfully until 35. Now I feel like I'm off the roller coaster. I also recognize that trauma could overwhelm me, but on a daily basis, my mood is much more even. I don't miss the ups and downs.

Antoine: I don't dream as much about what I can do, or what's going to happen, or something being a success—like writing this screenplay; I just work on it, and that's it. I don't think, Oh, it's going to be wonderful, or so-and-so is going to star in it. I just want it to be a tight, well-written mystery, with legitimate suspects and no holes in the story. As long as it's something I can be proud of, that's fine. If it doesn't go anywhere, at least I know it was a tight script.

Brian: My goals are more modest; I'm more satisfied with an ordinary life. In junior high I wanted to be president. I went to Yale Law School the year behind Bill Clinton. In my 30s, from time to time I regretted my decision to drop out of law school and join the Peace Corps. This usually happened when I was feeling vulnerable and unsure of myself. But I haven't felt that way in years, and I think that's a reflection of being more satisfied with my actual choices.

Hal: I don't get too grandiose anyway, but putting myself down has decreased. Success or failure doesn't mean anything about me; it's just part of the process. But I still have a difficult time with finances. If I don't have enough money, I get down on myself.

Steve: Work feels less vulnerable because I've already achieved something, so I don't feel so discouraged when I make a mistake or encounter a disappointment. However, I still feel pretty vulnerable to rejection in relationships.

I no longer assume that I'll be great. I made a few bricks we can use in building this wall, or cobblestones for the road. I can still entertain the fantasies, but now I see them as a pleasant daydream, instead of getting caught up in them. At midlife the infinite, numinous things become more concrete—like a gas cloud that becomes a planet. In youth I wanted to be a star. By midlife I'm satisfied being a planet—or maybe just an asteroid.

Wisdom and Reflection

As we age the grasping for glory, being the best, and conquering the world give way to a deeper appreciation of wisdom.

Perhaps grandiosity is needed when we're younger to sustain our initial efforts. We can understand this in terms of coming out—pride and a certain amount of self-righteousness can help us in our battles with homophobic families and institutions.

At midlife we may still feel very strongly about the same social issues that we cared about when we were younger. But we are often able to enlist more skillful means to make our point— partly because we no longer have to prove ourselves.

Wisdom often comes at the price of losing our innocence. We have a greater capacity for self-reflection and less need for self-deception. We have a more realistic sense of our own limitations and consequently a deeper empathy for others. Wisdom leads to a greater sense of modesty and equanimity.

Steve: I've studied a lot about midlife, so I'm familiar with these issues, but then I had to go through it myself. Now it's embodied wisdom. The experience of midlife moves from a thought to a scar. It's no longer a map, its a limp.

Mario: Patience is a virtue, and it's nice to have that. I'm the third oldest person in my company. I enjoy working with people in their 20s. I just went out to lunch with a coworker, and she was kind of rude to the waiter. She said she had no patience. I reminded her they could spit in your soup. That's wisdom.

Andrew: That's one of the biggest gifts of midlife. I have a very strong reflective side—about myself and about life. Because of that and my experience, I understand life and people a lot more. That brings a certain wisdom and serenity. I have a bigger picture, whereas before I was scrambling to figure it all out.

Tony: One of biggest things I am learning is that how people respond to me is often based on how I bring myself into a situation. The feeling I have about myself influences how others treat me. When I was younger and got whatever negative reaction I expected, I figured these people were just assholes—it's always them. It's only been the last few years that I've realized it's not just them—often it's not even them at all—it's me.

Hal: Wisdom is the balance between the heart and the mind, and I feel like I have that. Integrating thoughts and feelings, so neither one has the overriding vote on what happens.

Humor and Healing

The task for older men is not to be the hero but to be a healer.[13] Gay men are in a particularly advantageous place, as outsiders, to function as wounded healers, or shaman/tricksters for the larger society (see Chapter 10). A sense of humor helps us keep things in perspective, and we're less vulnerable to the ups and downs of everyday life.

Victor (Victor is 44 and Portuguese-American. He teaches a class on Buddhist psychology. He has a lover from Southeast Asia who is 16 years younger, and he shares his home with a longtime companion of 26 years): Having more perspective helps me realize that it doesn't help to infuse life with heaviness. The First Noble Truth: life is suffering. All these things are going to happen—death, illness, destruction—and at various times when it's not happening, it's cause for a party. This realization can infuse a range of things with some lightness.

Steve: During the rage stage of adjusting to my disability, nothing was humorous—nothing was funny. Now I feel like solar sails on a spaceship—sailing along instead of having to run my own engine. I find that I'm laughing at myself more. When I do stupid things or make mistakes, I used to get mad. Now I spill something and say, "Look at that mess—Steve must have been here."

Mario: Humor is so important in life. I listen to my siblings bickering, and I laugh at their squabbling. My mother says, "Why are you always laughing?" I watched David die; how can I take a jealous rivalry between my mother and sister seriously? They love me for it.

Hal: More than ever, I find myself laughing at situations. I laugh at myself, at how I see things going down. But behind that is some sadness that it shouldn't have to be that way. I've been on this healing path for 20 years. I wouldn't say I'm completely healed, but I have access to tools. If something powerful comes up, I know which tool to reach for.

Andrew: I can be a little obsessive, so my biggest challenge is about loosening up. Being in the moment, not being future-focused. When I'm in the moment, I can let go and feel the humor in the fullness of the moment. If I could do one thing that would be really good for me, that moment-to-moment awareness would be it.

Now that we've considered some of the strengths we bring to midlife, in the next chapter we'll look at some of the challenges we face during this transition.

Relating These Themes to Your Own Experience

For many men, midlife is a fairly introspective time. At the end of each chapter, I've included some thoughts and questions to help you relate these ideas to your own experience. You might want to keep a journal of your reactions, to keep track of feelings, memories, insights, and desires stimulated by these examples.

What positive aspects of midlife have you noticed in your own life?

If you like, draw a "life line" of your life up to this point, showing various milestones along the way, such as coming out, your first gay relationship, changes in your career, and other significant events.

Next, draw this line into the future, and mark in whatever new developments you'd like to see—all the way to the end.

What does this bring up for you?

Notes

1. A vivid example of sad resignation was portrayed by Andrew Holleran, author of *The Beauty of Men,* in a *New York Times Magazine* article called "The Wrinkle Room" (September 1, 1996). He suggested that loneliness is the destiny of gay men and that "gay geezers" are cast aside, "condemned to live out their days as forlorn relics taunted by memories of splendor." This was followed by a flurry of letters countering this attitude and affirming the self-worth of older gay men. Cited by Bruce Bawer in *The Advocate,* November 12, 1996, p. 96.
2. *Gay and Gray: The Older Homosexual Man* by Raymond M. Berger, p. 15. Urbana: University of Illinois Press, 1982.
3. *Male Homosexuals: Their Problems and Adaptations* by M.S. Weinberg and C.J. Williams. New York: Penguin, 1975.
4. "The Aging Male Homosexual: Myth and Reality" by J.J.

Kelly. *Gerontologist,* 17(4): pp. 328-32, 1977.

5. *Gay and Gray,* p. 184.

6. Ibid., p. 149.

7. "Growing Older Male: Heterosexual and Homosexual" by
    M.R. Laner. *Gerontologist,* 18(5): pp. 496-501, 1978.

8. A survey about age preferences for sexual contact was con-
    ducted by the Stop AIDS Project in San Francisco, with the
    following results:

    *   Of men in their 20s, 53% preferred older partners, while
        28% preferred those of the same age.

    *   77% of men in their 30s preferred partners the same age.

    *   34% of men in their 40s preferred partners the same age,
        and 47% preferred younger ones.

    *   Men in their 50s had evenly divided preferences: 42% pre-
        ferred partners the same age, and 42% preferred those who
        are younger.

    Results (based on 356 street interviews) presented at the Gen-
    eration Gap Community Forum, May 8, 1997, by the Stop
    AIDS Project, San Francisco. (I am aware of the "social ac-
    ceptability" bias of street interviews, but I think these results
    provide some initial impressions that could be explored by fur-
    ther research.)

9. See "Ability to Envision a Future Predicts Safe Sex Among
    Gay Men" by C. Frutchey, W. Blankenstein, and R. Stall.
    From the *Abstracts of the Ninth International Conference on
    AIDS,* June 1993, Berlin. Abstract PO-D06-3835. (Cited by
    Robert Kertzner. See note 3, Chapter 6.)

10. Stop AIDS Project, May 1997.

    *   41% of men in their 20s had positive things to say about
        growing older, such as "good" and "looking forward to it,"
        while 34% made negative statements.

* 57% of men in their 30s felt positive.
* 54% of men in their 40s had positive things to say, and
* 64% of men in their 50s felt positive about growing older.

11. *Gay and Gray,* p. 15.
12. *Beyond the Hero* by Allan Chinen, p. 89. New York: Tarcher/Putnam, 1993.
13. Ibid., p. 9.

CHAPTER 2

READY OR NOT!

A major task for gay men is coming to terms with our sexual orientation and figuring out how to thrive within a basically hostile and homophobic culture. The resolution of this task influences all later adjustments. Unresolved issues surrounding sexual orientation may be restimulated at midlife.

Just as we've finally arrived at a tightly knit sense of ourselves, usually by our mid to late 30s, it begins to unravel. In many ways midlife is like adolescence—previously repressed material breaks out, and whatever was left unfinished comes up again: conflicts over self-image, sexual attractiveness, beliefs, career goals, and confusion about how to connect with other men.

Developmental theories for men's changes at midlife often reflect heterosexual assumptions about what it means to be a man in our society. Gay men's response to the midlife transition has been neglected by most mainstream studies.[1] Results of gay oppression, such as lowered self-esteem and internalized homophobia, have been cited as evidence of homosexual pathology rather than being understood as the result of prejudice and dis-

crimination.[2] We need more research on this transition that ac-
knowledges the impact of homophobia, AIDS, and alternative
lifestyles on our development.[3] It's also helpful to recognize the
unique ways we have created gay relationships and support
within our community, especially in the face of a larger culture
that wishes we would simply disappear.

In this chapter we'll go over some common challenges that gay
men may experience during this time. Next we'll list some stages
we may go through to come to terms with midlife changes.

◆   Gay Midlife Challenges   ◆

Without the social support heterosexual couples usually take
for granted, gay men have been very creative in discovering a variety of ways to live our lives: We often cross age, race, and class
boundaries in our relationships; many of us maintain friendships
with former lovers; and we generally have fewer family restraints
if we decide to change career paths. Some of us have celebrated
our relationships with our own commitment ceremonies, and
others are adopting kids or coparenting with lesbian friends.
This freedom from heterosexual models can be liberating and
exciting, but it can also be disorienting, especially when we're
trying to assess where we've been and where we're going.

While this book focuses on gay men who came out as young
adults, the issues facing men who are just coming out at midlife
are usually compounded by a prolonged search for identity. They
experience many of the same challenges, but in the context of a
major restructuring of their self-image. This can include coming
out of a heterosexual marriage, dealing with the reactions of chil-

dren and relatives, and reevaluating occupational goals.[4]

Midlife is a time of increased introspection, which can eventually be a source of rich fulfillment: We get in touch with what's really important to us, and that can motivate us to make significant changes in our lives. In the beginning this self-examination can lead to doubt and anxiety. Yet once we get through this transition, many men report being much happier and more content than when they were younger.[5]

Confronted on all sides by apparent limitations (physical, sexual, and remaining time), at midlife we begin to reassess our priorities and possibilities. Let's look at how we can meet some of the following midlife challenges.

Midlife challenges:
- Depression and lethargy
- Disillusionment
- Distress over physical signs of aging
- Death anxiety/awareness of mortality

Depression and Lethargy

For some men, the realization that something has changed comes about gradually. It's not always experienced as a crisis, but over time, there's an increasing sense of dissatisfaction: Work may not seem as fulfilling as it once did, former interests begin to pale, or it's harder to get going with as much enthusiasm as we once had.

This feeling of lethargy can lead to depression, and it's difficult to envision new interests or goals. "Been there, done that" is a common complaint—it seems as though nothing really excites us anymore. There may be a sense of existential malaise—challenges feel like a burden instead of being invigorating.

Brian: In my late 40s I went into analysis because I felt as though my life was over and I was just waiting to die. I wasn't suicidal, but there was nothing new, so my notion of life was that you just go on until it ends. I would frequently wake up feeling unhappy—whatever made me happy before wasn't working, but I didn't know what else to do.

Mario: I have more independence, settling in my own way—that's been nice. But also some loneliness, since David died. Sometimes I feel lonely when the phone doesn't ring, but then when someone calls, I have nothing to say. I'm going back to therapy to deal with that. Waiting for Godot or to talk with someone—but then I don't know what to talk about.

Tony: I've always had some depression and lethargy, but that's actually lessening. My mother and brother also suffer from depression, and antidepressants have helped me a lot. I no longer spiral down the way I used to, and I can more easily stop a train of thought that's leading nowhere.

Andrew: I used to feel more depressed, but I don't anymore. I feel fuller inside because of my spiritual practice—having more internal satisfactions rather than looking outside for a sense of contentment. Partly because of all the therapy I've done, which has helped me become more self-accepting.

Disillusionment

Disillusionment includes a growing dissatisfaction in work, friends, and love. It often entails a loss of the feeling of omnipotence, as youthful ideals become tarnished—world peace, true love, becoming famous, or being a star no longer seem possible. And for those who have experienced great success, the triumphs of the past can seem strangely empty.

As we age, the blemishes on our heroes become more obvious, and the easy answers from former belief systems can no longer sustain us. But because we have established ourselves to some degree, we're not as dependent on outward authority for approval. This gives us the opportunity to develop our own internal sense of what is meaningful for us.

Tony: When I was young I believed that most of the anti-Communist messages we got were simply propaganda. I realized with the revolution in Eastern Europe in the late '80s that people really had been oppressed by those governments.

During the hippie era love, peace, and commitment were the ideals, but I saw many types of exploitation taking place there as well. I remember thinking Buddhism was the answer, or true Christianity versus organized religion, but then I met people who I respected, like monks from various traditions, and realized that they have problems too.

There are no easy answers. I no longer believe in sweeping change. Every system is flawed because humans run the system, and human beings are flawed. I now see that change is slow and incremental, and takes place a step at a time.

Hal: I get disillusioned because I see the possibilities, but the culture doesn't have a model for how they could be developed. I get discouraged when I see Bill Gates make $3 billion in 20 minutes. Our numbers get more and more skewed. I've had this impression since I was a kid, but now I have more years of evidence that this is weird.

We're more exposed, more out as gay people, yet even in the

Bay Area, gays are still being hassled. That will probably still exist for another 200 years. At midlife I've gained a broader perspective on social change and figure that's just what we have to deal with.

Randy: During my 40s I felt disillusioned with American society—especially after 12 years of Republican selfish, me-first, racist, homophobic, and holier-than-thou politics. Friends who tried to go into government during the '80s just lost out. I'm not a cockeyed optimist at this point—we're still building more prisons than schools—but I feel more hopeful now. I think the nation as a whole wants to try something different. I feel more of a sense of inclusiveness now than I have in many years.

Victor: My profession is not as I'd like it to be. Psychology under managed care is evolving in ways that seem unethical and uncaring. That's disillusioning.

In Buddhism the Second Noble Truth is that all suffering is caused by grasping. To the extent that I have a rigid vision of the way things are supposed to be, then I will suffer when things don't turn out that way. The alternative is to allow it to happen. So if I insist that all psychologists must always be ethical according to my definition, I can make myself miserable.

In my saner moments I can say these things—other times I'm grasping and enraged about how unfair the world is. In my saner moments I see that nothing is going to stay the way it is.

Andrew: On a spiritual level there's an increasing realization that the world doesn't offer me the fulfillment that I can get through my spiritual practice. I see the limitations of the world—and because I find a greater richness within myself, the impact isn't so powerful. The disillusionment is with the world, with the limitations of what it can offer, but I'm not in a disillusioned state.

Distress Over Physical Signs of Aging

The decline of youthful attractiveness can be very distressing, especially in a culture that seems to value sex appeal over all other qualities. If the kind of guy we find attractive doesn't age along with us, we can find ourselves drawn to men who are increasingly younger than we are—although, as the research cited in Chapter 1 indicates, this may be more stereotype than reality.

We also become more aware of physical limitations—we may not have quite the stamina we used to, either physically or sexually. It's easier to put on weight, and we need to be more conscientious about getting enough exercise. (We'll look at more examples of physical and sexual changes in Chapter 5.)

Randy: We've bought into the cultural ideal that we can remain ageless. Since I just turned 50, I'm aware of all these celebrities turning 50. Jane Fonda can still be sexy at 50; Hillary Clinton can still be with-it and attractive. I suppose part of it is celebrating the fact that we can feel and look healthier than our parents did at our age.

We're charting a new frontier of what it means to be middle-aged, even with all our liposuction and plastic surgery denial—but also in a healthy sense—we can dress in bright colors and have passionate sex even though we're 50 or 60. Maybe there's this underlying shadow, and we're just fooling ourselves. In our 60s we'll still be windsurfing and skateboarding. Will this attitude make it worse when we really hit old age?

Tony: I make a big deal about fading youth with my friends, but I'm fairly content with how I look. I do look at younger men with all their energy and excitement about life. They look beautiful, and I realize that those days are gone for me. I'm never going to have a body like that again.

Brian: Growing older, I've had to recognize that all cultures admire the beauty of youth. It's not just gay or Madison Avenue. Maybe we have an exaggerated image of youthful beauty, but smooth skin is beautiful, and young men are vibrant and alive. There is a certain beauty in aging, but the loss of one's beauty is just life, and that's OK.

Kevin: I wouldn't want to do my 20s or 30s over again. It would be nice to have the body, but not the angst. I know who I am, and I know much more about life—what's possible and what isn't. I've lived long enough to see that shit happens and you go on.

Death Anxiety/Awareness of Mortality

The first part of adulthood is often spent on establishing oneself. It's a time of expansion and growth and increasing opportunities. But gradually this sense of expansiveness is displaced by an awareness of limitations. We may fear that time will run out before we've had the chance to really live or accomplish anything momentous. At midlife we also become more conscious of our own mortality. Aging parents may be ailing or dying, and becoming increasingly dependent.

For gay men, this consciousness has been forcefully brought home because of AIDS. Although there is a new hopefulness due to recent advances in treatments, the overwhelming loss we've experienced has made us acutely aware of our own mortality. (We'll look at more examples of dealing with mortality in Chapter 8.)

Victor: I don't experience my awareness of death as anxiety. I'm aware that I've been here 44 years, and I extrapolate that forward—I'll be very old at 88 and thinking a lot more about death. I'm aware of the fact that this body is not going to live forever at another level, now, not just intellectually. I had this feeling in my 20s that I had all the time in the world, with un-limited possibilities. The possibilities still feel unlimited, but not time.

Kevin: I know from watching friends die that even death is generally doable. For the first time in my life I'm capable of to-tally relaxing. There's just a lot of peace in knowing who you are, and it takes a lot of time to get there. Maybe some men in their 20s have it easier. It's nice to know I could leave the world tomorrow and not really have any regrets.

Brian: Solve this midlife puzzle: Live for the moment, but there's so much to do! There are too many interesting people and more good, worthwhile things to do than there is time to do them in. I find myself wrestling with this paradox. My mother has time but not enough energy. The other day I saw a young man just sitting by the ocean, reminding me of my youth. But now I don't have time to just take a day and sit by the ocean and daydream.

◆ Stages ◆

This sense of unease, disillusionment, and limitation can leave us rather downcast about our prospects. Men react in various ways to these changes and feelings—some may simply try hard-er, while others try to evade them. (We'll explore types of evasion in the next chapter.) In the end most of us manage to come to terms with these changes and even make the best of them.

Now let's look at some common midlife stages, to see how these characteristics may express themselves during this transition:[6]

Overview of midlife stages:
- Restlessness
- Trying harder
- It doesn't work
- Allowing uncertainty
- Letting go
- Opening to new possibilities
- Integrating changes

Restlessness

Feeling restless is related to the depression and lethargy noted above. There's a sense of meaninglessness—previous interests just don't have the same pull anymore. You may also feel anxiety over lost opportunities, and it seems as though the world is passing you by. There's a sense of urgency, but without any clear direction, it's easy to feel out of sorts, irritable, and agitated.

Brian: I realized I was depressed when I made what I thought was an offhand comment to a friend: "Life is busier and busier but emptier and emptier." I thought it didn't bother me; it was simply true, not that heavy. I can see now that my restlessness was a manifestation of a deeper depression and dissatisfaction.

Trying Harder

This sense of restlessness may lead to an impulse to do something, anything, just to break the tension. At first you may simply try harder—by throwing yourself back into work, for example, or by trying something new—taking up a new sport, buying a new car, or dating a new boyfriend. There's nothing wrong with trying to take better care of ourselves, and sometimes a major change in job, locale, or love interest makes a lot of sense. But change for its own sake in this early stage often has an impulsive, quick-fix quality about it.

The idea is to be able to tolerate these feelings and look for the true meaning of our restlessness and dissatisfaction. Rather than acting immediately just to get away from this agitated state, staying with this process can eventually provide us with a clear direction.

Antoine: The thought came up for me of trying harder—but I just seemed to make messes. Doing stuff at the office, I would miss a lot of things by not being careful. I prefer to do things well. I want to do a lot, but I don't want to leave garbage behind.

Mario: I have a lot more tolerance for my feelings. If I'm depressed, I'm willing to sit and let it reveal itself to me, rather than acting right away or having a drink.

It Doesn't Work

We try to assuage our restlessness by using what we're familiar with. We may feel initially gratified, but simply doing more of the same, rededicating ourselves, or trying harder doesn't really satisfy us. The reason this quick fix doesn't work is that it's usually not in tune with the yearning for a deeper significance that is growing within us. We still feel empty, but we're at a loss as to what else to do.

Hal: I thought I needed to do something different, better, or more—but it didn't work. I just saw the results weren't consistent with the amount of effort I was putting in.

Allowing Uncertainty

Instead of doing something impulsive in order to alleviate our anxiety, what we really need is time to reflect. By allowing ourselves a period of "not knowing," we can get in touch with the deeper stirrings inside us that may lead to a new direction. We can pay attention to dreams, use a journal to explore different possibilities, sort through our options in therapy, and not have to act right away.[7]

Hal: That's what I do. Like a meditation, just to say if this works out, fine. But it applies to other things too, being with a partner, say, or even taking a lane in traffic.

Victor: The place of not knowing—the only thing we can do during this stage is simply to be in that place. This is difficult to do, especially in this culture where we're seduced by the belief that our ego can do anything. Just work harder, and everything will be all right. It's important to remind ourselves that this is the voice that's creating the discomfort. It's fine to be in between—neither here nor there. We need to create more support for that in our culture.

Andrew: Uncertainty—this is the stage where I am at the moment. There are some changes I want to make that are pretty scary, like taking some time off or even changing careers. I'm not sure if I can pull it off logistically. It would be a radical change.

Letting Go

During this time we begin to let go of our previous self-image, recognize our mistakes and feel our regrets. We can come to terms with the past by developing a sense of compassion for ourselves and others. This allows us to be open to new growth and development, rather than simply trying to compensate for previous mistakes or make up for lost time.

Victor: Early identity formation takes a lot of work, and once we've got one we have to defend it. But as we get older, that identity becomes frayed, and it's time to do something new.

Opening to New Possibilities

A tentative vision may lead to exploring new interests, but without the impulsive desire to escape from our restlessness that we experienced earlier. Instead, a gradual sense of clarity develops within us. We try out a few different possibilities to see how they fit and eventually settle on a new direction.

Victor: Midlife is like adolescence. There's a new awakening—anything seems possible again, though not in terms of time. My sense of people who negotiate this transition the best are those who are willing to go for broke. Just deal with whatever shows up—that's really incredible—all these urges and new stuff showing up—the trick is how to be in the world with all this new material.

It may be a lot quieter than adolescence, but it's no less powerful. What's happening is a whole new constellation in identity. Those parts that are emerging now were left unchosen because they conflicted with an earlier self-image. But that just means they're more complex. And when they show up again with an extra 20 years of experience, that can be an incredible adventure!

I was very introverted when I was younger. I would never go to parties; I'd give a paper and then leave a professional conference rather than stick around and socialize. But over the last few years, I've gotten much more in touch with my extroverted side. This part of me came along that I didn't even know was there, and it's a lot of fun.

Integrating Changes

By integrating these changes into the rest of our lives, we can feel more secure about our potential for continuing growth. We can then embark on our new direction with increasing confidence. For example, I had a client who had neglected his interest in art because it was put down as effeminate by his father when he was a kid. But the more he pushed it away, the more depressed he became, until he finally admitted that he still wanted to express himself artistically. Then he needed to overcome the belief that he couldn't express himself in this way un-

less he was a great artist or at least "talented." Finally he realized he enjoyed the process of creation, regardless of whether he
could make a living at it or be considered "great" by anyone else.
This is an example of the shift from outward standards to an internal sense of meaning and self-worth.

Hal: I see midlife as the end of assimilation and digestion, the
end of introspection and self-absorption—now it's more about
the outside. In the past I've been working on myself, and now
it's more about putting out what I've assimilated. Right now I'm
in this growth phase of expansion. That feels the strongest—on
shaky ground, still, or a shaky branch, but that feels like where
I'm headed.

◆   Soaring, Crashing, Walking   ◆

For some, this sense of restlessness or unease may come
about as a natural development at midlife—we're simply ready
to try something new or recapture neglected aspects of ourselves. But a crisis in self-identity can also be instigated by a
major loss. By our late 30s, everything seems to be going along
fine, when disaster strikes—through an accident, a physical
disability, a layoff, an illness, or a major disappointment. Our
whole notion of reality is upended: Our previous identity is
jeopardized, our sense of meaning destroyed, and we're thrown
into despair.

Yet out of that despair can come some new growth, because
we're being challenged to develop another part of ourselves that
had previously lain dormant. By reaffirming the importance of
an earlier goal, we may be willing to sacrifice everything else to-

ward that end. In a similar way, many gay men with HIV have been forced to reevaluate what's really important to them. Following is an example of these stages through Steve's experience with a number of significant losses:

Steve: Things were going along fine in love and work—then disaster struck, and everything fell apart. First I had the break-up with my lover, then I didn't get a major research grant, and later I developed carpal tunnel syndrome, so I could no longer type. I found myself wandering in the dark, raging against fate, and then gradually coming out of it. Midlife for me can be summarized as soaring, crashing, and then walking.

Trying harder

I tried everything I could think of to deal with the pain in my hands. I've spent more money on physical therapy, doctors, and prosthetics than on anything else.

It doesn't work

I went to all kinds of specialists, but nothing seemed to work. My hands didn't get better. I felt rage and despair. During my rage phase, I threw things and even broke a computer keyboard. I thought, *You'll never get better, so why even try.* I felt like giving up, with apathy and despair.

Allowing uncertainty

I lost everything—my household, my partner, my career, my health. The path ran out in the direction I was traveling, with no clear trail ahead. I found myself wandering in the darkness.

Letting go

I had to let go of certain expectations and beliefs:

I won't ever be able to type or write fast again.

I couldn't swim because of the problems with my hands and started to get a potbelly.

Letting go of hopes of growing older with my lover.

Letting go of being pain-free.

The hardest part for me was letting go of the known and tolerating the anxiety of what was coming next. But I also found myself letting go of conventionality or caring what other people think or always trying to do the right thing. For a while I found myself eating chocolates, watching soap operas, and self-indulging just to lighten things up.

Even though part of me wanted to give up, I also wanted to resist. Like with doing research—even though I could no longer type, I wouldn't give it up. I felt stubborn. This crisis forced me to develop a clearer sense of what was important to me. So I let go of things that seemed less important, like swimming, in order to keep things that were crucial, like research and writing.

In youth I had this romantic notion of sacrificing everything for the sake of exploring these ideas—even being a starving artist. Now hopefully it won't come to that, but if it does, it does. Part of disillusionment is realizing it doesn't all come out like you hoped it would.

Opening to new possibilities

Now I'm asking other people for help and depending on them in ways I never did before. I'm also spending more for fun, extravagant stuff, like extra vacations. I see my own self-indulgence coming out of the fact that I've had to suffer so much, I want some dessert.

Integrating changes

My work recrystallized around research, which has always been essential for me. Also, integrating at a lower level of intensity. Before I could go at warp drive. Now I go more slowly, less on impulse.

We've looked at common themes and stages of the midlife transition, and as we can see with Steve's example, it doesn't always go that smoothly. A lot of gay men experience these impending changes with a certain amount of dread, resistance, and denial. In the next chapter we'll look at some of the pitfalls of denial at midlife, when some gay men try to escape from these tasks and become "lost in the dark wood."

Relating These Themes to Your Own Experience:

- What are some of the challenges you have faced at midlife?
- Mark these on your time line.
- How have you tried to deal with setbacks and disappointments?
- What stages have you found yourself going through in response to these changes?

Notes

1. See "Middle Adulthood in the Theories of Erikson, Gould, and Vaillant: Where Does the Gay Man Fit?" by C.W. Cornett and R.A. Hudson. They discuss the relevance of various midlife theories to gay male issues. *Journal of Gerontological Social Work,* 10 (3/4), pp. 61-73.

A major study of men in general, *The Seasons of A Man's Life*
by D.J. Levinson (New York: Knopf, 1978), had only one page
with two examples of men dealing with homosexuality, and
both men tried to go straight. Nonetheless, Levinson provides
a helpful outline of male development, and he divides midlife
into four stages:

* Settling down and becoming one's own man (33–40):
Seeking stability, security, and comfort, and actively carving
out one's niche in society—"I want to make my place in
this world."

* Middle transition (40–45): Assessment of accomplishments
and development of another life structure—"What is it I really want?"

* Midlife (45–50): Accepting one's fate—"What I have
achieved is OK."

* Age 50, transition, and midlife culmination (50–60):
Finding security and self-acceptance—"What I have become
is OK."

2. "Heterosexual Bias in Psychological Research on Lesbianism
    and Male Homosexuality" by S. Morin in *American Psycholo-
    gist*, 32, pp. 629-637. Also "Gay Male Identities: Concepts
    and Issues" by John C. Gonsiorek in *Lesbian, Gay, and Bisex-
    ual Identities Over the Lifespan*, edited by A.R. D'Augelli and
    C.J. Patterson, p. 29. New York: Oxford University Press, 1995.

3. "Lavender and Gray: A Brief Survey of Lesbian and Gay
    Aging Studies" by Margaret Cruikshank in *Gay Midlife and
    Maturity*, edited by John Alan Lee. New York: Haworth
    Press, 1991.

Many of these studies dealt with men who came of age before
the Stonewall rebellion. It would be helpful to have some longitudinal studies, which follow a group of gay men through

out their lives; time-lag studies, comparing age groups from different historical periods (for example, comparing men reached midlife during the '70s with those who reached midlife during the '90s); and cohort studies, which would look at the specific times that groups of men went through each stage of development. By looking at midlife from these different angles, we could compare whether the changes gay men experience at midlife reflect coming of age during a particular historical time or whether these are common reactions for gay men at midlife across the decades. Comparing class, ethnicity, and philosophical or spiritual beliefs would also help round out the picture of how gay men fare at midlife. Other suggestions for further research are included in Kimmel and Sang, p. 209 (see note 4).

For examples of the impact of homophobia on gay identity, see *Being Homosexual: Gay Men and Their Development* by Richard Isay. New York: Farrar, Straus, and Giroux, 1989.

4. "Lesbians and Gay Men in Midlife" by D.C. Kimmel and B.E. Sang. *In Lesbian, Gay, and Bisexual Identities Over the Lifespan,* p. 202. For a description of coming out later in life, see *Uncharted Lives: Understanding the Life Passages of Gay Men* by Stanley Siegel and Ed Lowe Jr. New York: Dutton, 1994.

5. "Theories of the Male Midlife Crisis" by O.G. Brim in *The Counseling Psychologist,* 1976, pp. 2-9.

6. I developed these stages from various theories in the developmental literature as well as my own observations and interviews with clients, colleagues, and the men in these interviews. As with any stage theory, it's useful to see this as descriptive of some men's experience rather than prescriptive of what you "should" be experiencing.

7. In his book *In Midlife,* Murray Stein provides an extensive description of this uncertain place, which he calls the "liminal" phase. He uses Greek myths to provide a Jungian perspective on midlife. Dallas: Spring Publications, 1983.

CHAPTER 3

INTO THE DARK WOOD

Midway through life's journey, I went astray from the straight road and found myself lost in a dark wood.
—Dante, *Divine Comedy*

The "dark wood" that Dante refers to in the opening lines of *Divine Comedy* can be understood as a place of psychic uncertainty. We are betwixt and between—no longer young men gadding about the gay community, footloose and fancy-free. We suddenly find ourselves looking in, outsiders once again. This whole transition can be terribly unsettling. Without a clear sense of what it means to be a gay man at midlife, we may feel insecure in our new identity, confused, lost, and wandering.

Yet the uncertainty that accompanies this transition may seem familiar to gay men. Most of us left the "straight road" behind when we acknowledged our homosexuality to ourselves, our families, and to the world. By the time we reach midlife, we've usually accomplished a lot, challenging the effects of discrimination and oppression, and countering our own internalized homophobia.

In this chapter we'll look at the task of reaching closure with a youthful identity. Then we'll examine the pitfalls of denial at midlife, when some gay men are tempted to escape from having to deal with these changes and lose themselves in the dark wood.

◆   Reaching Closure With a Youthful Identity   ◆

At midlife we gradually separate from our former identity as a boy or a younger man. This doesn't mean that we give up youthful attitudes or aspirations, such as keeping ourselves fit and active. But we recognize that a shift is taking place within us. We begin to reassess possibilities in the face of personal limitations. As we become more aware of the passing of youth, our sense of self is no longer so largely determined by how others see us. We develop more of an internal sense of self-reflection and definition. At the end of this process, we emerge from that place of "betwixt and between" with a new identity. No longer impetuous youths, we begin to take our place among the wiser elders.[1]

Kevin: I have let go of youthful visions of what my life would be. Although, when I was young, I never bothered wondering what my future would be. I was quite occupied with the moment.

Hal: I feel like I'm closing off the old identity and opening a whole new chapter of being a kid. Being childlike rather than being childish. Approaching life with a beginner's mind, fresh again.

Andrew: I feel youthful inside—in terms of my optimism in life. Balancing that with being 48 and the fact that I'm not a kid anymore. I still want someone to play with.

Randy: I think I reached closure with my own youthful identity some years ago—partly when I came out to my mother. Coming out to her enabled me to validate my identity as a gay man. She began to understand that this is who I am—not the boy she idealized me to be. And I no longer felt compelled to live out her image of what I was supposed to be.

Brian: I still have the same identity I had as a youth—that's still part of me—but I've got to move on. I've outgrown my identity as a youthful person. I'm among the oldest 5% in a bar, and that doesn't feel like a comfortable place to be.

At midlife the question is no longer "What do I want to be when I grow up?" It's "What do I want to have accomplished before I die?" I have my career, friends and relationships, travels, all of which I started in my youth. Now I also want to be a good father who will have a positive impact on his son.

Tony: I went through a period where I wanted to be hip by dressing like a young man—with baggy shorts, a tank top, and black tennis shoes—stuff you don't usually see on a 45-year-old man.

In retrospect I realize that I wanted to be young again. I still wear comfortable clothes, but I don't feel it's age-inappropriate anymore. I won't wear a turned-around baseball cap or pierce my nose because it seems like something a 20-year-old would do. But I'll dress in ways I think look good.

There's not a certain way to be middle-aged. I used to think there was. You can be older and still be conscious about how you dress. I can wear a business suit and then go to the gym wearing baggy shorts—not trying to look younger than I am or be younger than I am—it just feels natural.

◆ Types of Evasion ◆

Even though we've been through a major life change before, when we came out as gay, we may not relish going through another one. We may be tempted to evade our fate—especially since our image of what it means to be a gay man at midlife in this culture has not been very appealing.

We can understand denial of changes at midlife as an attempt to shore up our previous self-image. This is a normal response to the anxiety brought about by physical, sexual, and emotional changes. It's tempting to return to a previous mode of functioning because it feels familiar. Yet this attempt to hold on to our youthful self-image usually doesn't work because it doesn't fit our current station in life. When we look at it objectively, it becomes increasingly obvious that we've outgrown it.

Gay men are incredibly creative, and we've developed various ways to avoid midlife. Unfortunately, our attempts at evasion usually sink us deeper into the quagmire and keep us from coming to terms with the demands of our true selves. Let's look at some common strategies of avoidance, and then we'll examine more effective ways of dealing with these changes.

Types of evasion:
- Making up for lost time
- Peter Pan
- Running amok
- Going down in flames
- Bitter queen

Making Up for Lost Time

During this uncertain time, when we've "lost our way," there may be a sense of not having accomplished anything. It may be difficult to remember earlier goals or to ascribe any significance to them. It's also hard to imagine what else we'd like to do. Rather than tolerating the anxiety of not knowing, some men are tempted to make up for lost time—through some radical change for its own sake or a mad dash to reclaim youthful ambitions. This tendency can also be compared to the stage of "bargaining" in grief reactions. If only I just work harder, exercise more, go to bars, get laid, buy a tank top, get a face lift, pierce my nipple, get a tattoo, or dye my hair—I'll be all right.

Hal: I see this all the time—older guys buy the red sports car—and gay men also do that by getting a younger lover. They take in some 20-year-old and then wonder why the relationship doesn't work.

Mario: I have a friend who hadn't had sex for years, and now he can't keep it in his pants.

Peter Pan

Gay men in general are often dismissed as delayed adolescents, boys who refuse to grow up and take on adult responsibilities. Yet many of our heterosexual friends envy the flexibility we have in various aspects of our lives—taking vacations, starting a new career, moving, or changing partners without going through wrenching divorces and child custody disputes.

If we don't have kids, what difference does it make if we live for the moment?

The danger of holding on to *puer eternus,* or eternal youth, is not in our refusal to conform to heterosexual norms. Rather, the danger lies in ascribing our sense of self-worth to youthful values and attributes that inevitably fade. If we put youth on a pedestal, when that pedestal eventually crumbles, so does our self-image.

"Party boy" culture is probably the most obvious example—pumping up with steroids at the gym, abusing alcohol and drugs, dancing all night, and having interchangeable sex partners. Of course, dancing the night away can be a lot of fun. It's only a problem if we assume that's all there is—indulging in sex and drugs but fleeing intimacy—because we don't know what else is possible. When we can no longer compete, the party's over, and it seems like nothing's left.

Kevin: I know a man who's 37, still doing the party circuit. He takes drugs and is very sexually active. He doesn't know what to do with companionship and sex. His values are changing, but I don't think he has a vision of what he wants in terms of love.

Hal: People say my youthful nature is what's most appealing about me. I still feel innocent, I think, because I have a beginner's mind. Refusing to be responsible, that's the negative side. I've wanted someone else to take responsibility, but no one's going to do it for me. Now I'm taking care of all the details of my life, whereas before I might have left it to others. Asking for help is fine, as opposed to waiting for someone to help me because they see me falling down.

Brian: I don't need things to be clarified or completed. I like to keep my options open and have trouble committing to things. Sometimes this gets me into trouble. I let phone calls go; I have a difficult time making decisions. Keeping my options open isn't really effective anymore because I no longer have unlimited options.

This youthful tendency has a positive side because it keeps me feeling vibrant and alive. I feel open to newness and change and flux. The challenge is to commit and stay steady and get settled in parts of life but also stay open and flexible. How to contain the youthful energy without squelching it—integrate it, not kill it off.

Victor: I still dance all night. Dancing has gone through many transitions with me. I was totally out of touch with my body when I was young. Dancing was a completely foreign idea—the idea of dancing in front of people horrified me.

I came out during the disco era, so I started going dancing and enjoyed it. It was a total epiphany that I could have a relationship with my body. Then dancing became a vehicle for meeting people. Most of the people I know I've met on the dance floor—whether for casual sex, friends, or a relationship. I'm not sure in the beginning how much dancing came out of my need to connect and how much was the pure pleasure of movement. But once I discovered my body could move, I didn't want to stop.

I recognize my dancing mania isn't really acting my age, but I don't care. I think it's actually very healthy. If the *puer* takes over, you're in trouble, but if the old fart takes over, you're in trouble too.

Andrew: Part of me stays a boy inside in terms of my curiosity and enthusiasm. I'm also very aware that I'm a man—it's sort of an inner attitude, rather than trying to maintain a certain status or look. I don't see this as a *puer* thing; I think of it as a way to go through life. I don't see myself as a boy; I see myself as a man, but I have a youthful attitude. I do see some men who stay stuck in that 30s culture. They don't grow into their age.

Steve: I think there's a positive side to *puer* and even to temporary evasion. It's playful and spontaneous, and it can be invigorating to indulge our youthful impulses. It's more a question of balance. My boyfriend was a Peter Pan. He left me after eight years and moved to Paris with a man he had just met.

Running Amok

The encounter with limitations at midlife can lead to the demise of youthful dreams and possibilities. Unless we have an image of another way to live that's promising and appealing, it's easy to succumb to the temptation of self-indulgence for as long as it lasts. This sense of uncertainty can lead to the desire to escape, not only by clinging to youthful images and ideals but also through self-destructive indulgence.

Of course we've all heard of the middle-aged married man who dumps his wife and runs off with his secretary. This is a common stereotype of how heterosexual men can be tempted to cope with a midlife crisis. Because we don't have many models for aging gracefully, this sort of reactive rebellion is also a danger for gay men.

Dumping a long-term partner, having affairs to prove our attractiveness, or quitting a job abruptly rather than developing a plan for changing one's career can all be seen as reactive changes brought about by a crisis in self-image. Running amok can be understood as an attempt to resolve the ambiguity we face in ways that seem familiar. It's motivated by a desire to escape from the discomfort of loss and change. The challenge is to stand aside and experience impulses without having to act on them immediately. Then we can make more conscious decisions rather than be driven by our impulses.

Mario: I find that more in younger men in their 30s, working the whole circuit scene, taking drugs, and striving for a buffed gym body. Running as fast as they can to fulfill this gay image propagated by our own culture. Still trying to be 25. I say, Slow down, honey, you've got a long ways to go.

They're paying for it by losing their looks prematurely, burning out on drugs and alcohol. A 29-year-old friend of mine just became HIV-positive. I asked him, "Who have you been with?" He said, "You. And this other guy—I don't know his name. I met him hiking out by Land's End." They had unprotected sex.

Hal: I see guys starting to use crack at 40, smoking Cuban cigars, and drinking fine champagne. They have the money now, so they want to have all the best stuff. Because they're not getting whatever it is they really need, they think more of these luxuries will make up the difference. Building up their bodies with steroids, using electrolysis, it's all for love, affection, for someone who will be there—for someone younger to say you're all right.

Victor: Running amok is often a breakthrough experience. For some people, that may just be what you have to pass through. You have to act it out before you can be aware of the fact that there are certain aspects you have repressed. Sometimes you have to have the consequences in your face before you can consciously see them and deal with them.

I knew a man who worked for a government bureaucracy. He was respected, had a nice home. But he started acting out these uncontrollable urges. He made some messes, like coming to work late, arguing with his boss, and coming on to his assistant, who already had a boyfriend. Fortunately, none of these was so messy he wasn't able to clean it up.

He couldn't stand being a prisoner of bureaucracy. He realized what he really wanted was to move to a resort and open a bed and breakfast in his 50s, so that's what he did. He wouldn't have let himself know he was dissatisfied if these unconscious urges hadn't forced him to act out to get his attention. This was not some demonic part of his personality—it was simply doing the only thing it could do to shake him out of his rut. This part of him had tried to get his attention in more subtle ways, like being bored or dissatisfied, but he kept plodding along until he got grabbed by the collar and shaken by the mess he'd gotten himself into.

Mario: I still run amok every now and then. It comes in flurries. It's the game of the '80s that I learned: Can I walk up to a young man who's attractive and bring him home? It's a sense of validation. Then I try to pursue the friendship part, and it doesn't work. He says, "You're 42; you're my father's age," then I never see him again.

Brian: Some running amok is reactive but still healthy. It can get you in touch with what's really missing. I've also seen guys using drugs and going to dance clubs past the age where it's satisfying. It feels empty—you ask, "Why am I doing this?" Then you realize you're really not getting your needs met. This might have worked when I was 25—it's great to lose myself in the crowd, with all the movement, the whirling mass of flesh. I see it as a developmental phase, but some hang on too long. Drugs, sex, and rock and roll—one thing about getting older—you get tired and just can't do it anymore.

Going Down in Flames

As young gay men we may have the illusion that we could party forever without any real connections, because it may not occur to us that anything else is even possible. The avoidance of commitment may not even be conscious. A fear of intimacy may derive from earlier rejections and homophobic attacks. At the same time we have few images of what it means to be an older gay man and still be seen as desirable or having anything to offer.

For some men, the idea of the party ending (at least as we've known it) seems intolerable. In response to the crisis of aging, it's not a question so much of acting out. It's more like a purposeful rejection of moderation, a reveling in extreme self-indulgence—unsafe sex, drugs, even trouble with the law—an apparently romantic desire to go down in flames.

Some men would rather die than give up the dream of eternal youth. The myth of Icarus, who flew so close to the sun that his wings melted and he plunged to his death, provides a telling image of this sacrifice to the gods of youthful self-indulgence. These men end by flaming out, not caring about the consequences—maybe even welcoming them—partly because they can't imagine life after 40 anyway.

Mario: The friend who's sexually active again is also an incredible alcoholic. He got so drunk I was embarrassed, to say nothing of scared shitless the way he was driving like a maniac. I told him I would never go out with him again. We sit and talk at home; that's fine, but I'm not going out with him when he's getting trashed.

I still do drugs now and then, like mushrooms. But it's a

planned event, with boundaries, not like taking LSD and then going to a dance club. I haven't done that in years. If I did, it would be out in the woods with a couple of friends. The younger men I know do it all the time. They take ecstasy and speed twice a week and say they don't have a problem. But I can see the paranoia, the jitters, the denial—it's sad. The risky behavior is really sad.

A couple I know recently broke up. Being friends with both, I tried not to get in the middle, but both were talking to me. Finally I got them together and said, "You two need to talk about what's going on." They were having unsafe sex—one is positive, and the other is negative. It was the drugs that got them into unsafe sex. Fortunately, the other guy still tested negative.

The reason for the breakup was the unsafe sex, brought on by the drugs. I told the one who was HIV-positive that I wanted to slap him, how could he put his lover at risk? And the other guy, how could you be such a dope? Yet I love them too.

It's unfortunate when I meet someone my age who's out of touch with the ability to communicate. You have to communicate about what's going on and learn to listen. Not many gay men have those skills.

Bitter Queen

The "bitter queen" is a stereotype—albeit a homophobic one—that gay men frighten each other with. It probably represents our own worst fear of what we might become: a fussy, demanding, cynical queen who projects his own avarice and jaundiced views onto everyone else but has a hard time seeing that it's coming from him.

Understanding this stereotype as a form of internalized homophobia can help us realize that we all may have a bit of the bitter queen inside us. We've all been hurt by other men—our fathers, brothers, bullies—and even by other gay men, who have used us, abused us, or disillusioned us.

Part of the problem is that we may still be comparing ourselves to earlier standards, but we can no longer compete. We disdain anyone who aspires to these unrealistic goals, but we may also secretly envy them. Without a vision of what else is possible—if we haven't come up with anything to replace being a hunk or a party boy—we may be tempted to tear others down or disparage them with sour grapes ("Just who does she think she is!"). Of course, many of us never identified with being a hunk or a party boy when we were younger, either. By comparing ourselves to unrealistic models or a narrow range of media-created images, we can feel left out, isolated, and angry.

Older gay men in our culture lack a sense of "place." With no recognized role (other than this negative one), it's easy to end up feeling cast aside and estranged, like Bette Davis in *All About Eve.* Our image of the bitter queen is no doubt a reflection of society's sexism, but it can also be understood as our own worst fear: to become "feminized" in a devouring, bitter, and castrating way. We need to find our own ways to express authority without becoming a tyrannical, bitchy queen.

The choice here is between contempt and generativity—finding a way to make a contribution rather than wallowing in our own disappointments and becoming disdainful of others. The contempt is prompted by despair, loneliness, and grief. It's usually a reflection of our own internalized homophobia and the contempt we feel toward ourselves.

Contempt can be understood as an early reaction to grief. We recognize the loss of our previous self-image, but we don't yet know what else can take its place. We can replace this bitterness by first acknowledging our losses and grieving for the actual changes we face physically, sexually, and socially. Then we can create a new place (and status) for ourselves within the gay community that provides us with a sense of meaning, respect, and purpose. But this can only happen by treating each other (and ourselves) with the same level of respect and consideration that we wish we had from younger men.

Some older men are resistant to being recognized or labeled as "elders." They don't want "respect" in the sense of being seen as different, even if it means being exalted in some way, because it separates them from others. Demanding respect or putting ourselves on a pedestal is not the answer. It's more of a shift in our own attitude that can lead us to redefining what it means to be an older gay man in our culture.

Victor: One of my closest friends became bitter before he died. We will all get old and sick and die. That's what suffering is—a very primary thing, and it's the hardest thing to accept. He couldn't stand that he was no longer other men's sexual fantasy. All these parties and sexual adventures were going on around him, and he was no longer invited to participate. He was so angry at everyone and everything, he became inaccessible because he was so bitter. I could no longer talk to him about it. It's an example of holding on to the dream of what life was supposed to be like forever, rather than accepting what was happening in the moment.

Brian: It's the gay version of a conservative curmudgeon, who can't keep his heart open to change. He hasn't worked through the loss, so he becomes bitter about everything. When I see a cute young man, sometimes I feel like a bitter old queen. I feel an impulse to do something absurd, like throwing myself at him or trying to seduce him. When we're not getting our desires met, it's easy to feel contempt, which is really a disguised form of loss and desire.

Andrew: I have a couple of friends who are growing older and just figure they're going to be alone. One feels a lot of loss and the other a lot of bitterness disguised as resignation.

When he talks about it, he has a lot of anger in his voice. And under that is a sense of hurt about not being responded to or loved in the way he thinks he should be. I can get bitter once in a while by the fact that I'm not paid attention to. "Men are pigs" sorts of comments come to mind. But I try not to dwell there.

Tony: A friend of mine was really good-looking, got cruised all the time when he was younger. Now he's 40, and that just doesn't happen anymore. I wouldn't say he's bitter, but it's been hard for him to adjust to.

Steve: Window-shopping and looking at young men could go either way—sometimes I feel like an appreciative audience, but other times I feel bitter and envious, disdainful and contemptuous.

◆   Recovery at Midlife   ◆

As one might expect, the challenges we face at midlife can be exacerbated for men in recovery from alcohol and substance abuse. Even with fairly stable recovery, it can be tempting to use again in the face of disappointments, confusion, isolation, and a loss of self-esteem. It's essential to reach out for support during this time, so you don't succumb to using again as a way to avoid midlife challenges. We don't have to be overwhelmed by these changes; mutual support can make our journey through the dark wood seem more like a shared adventure. Having support makes us less likely to act out our unease by using, with all its well-known dangers and complications (like running amok, flaming out, or becoming bitter).[2]

Tony: Whether it was alcohol, religion, or sex, I kept hoping something outside of myself would make my life easier—it would take away the pain, the disillusionment, and help me feel better. Now I realize that I need to focus on taking care of myself rather than getting distracted by these tempting escapes. I may still feel a lack of confidence at times, but I know that trying to bolster my self-esteem by using drugs, alcohol, or sex is only going to make things worse.

◆   Coming Out of the Darkness   ◆

The current crisis may seem like our last chance to really accomplish something momentous—we may be tempted to move, to leave a relationship, to start a new career. There's nothing wrong with wanting to look our best, accomplish our goals, and take care of our bodies. And it may be that a major shift in our lives is exactly what we need. But change for its own sake can be a way to distract ourselves from the larger questions we face at this juncture of our lives. So how do we tell the difference?

If we allow ourselves some time in the dark wood to take

stock of ourselves, we're less likely to dash off madly in all directions. It's the desperate attempt to hold on to a youthful image that gets us into trouble—eventually the youthful mask falls away, and we're horrified by the remaining portrait of Dorian Gray.

During this transition we often find ourselves walking a tightrope between running amok and repression. We may be tempted toward wild ventures to escape from uncertainty. Leaping to a solution is an attempt to avoid our anxiety rather than sitting with it. We tend to see an external change as the answer, whereas the "answer" may reveal itself through an internal shift in perspective.

In contrast, a loving self-acceptance can also motivate us to take care of ourselves, reevaluate our goals, and make decisions about our future—but in a way that's healing and full of growth rather than self-defeating or unrealistic.

As mentioned earlier, this conscious quest will not necessarily be smooth sailing—there will be plenty of soul-searching, questioning, and doubt—but it's better to tolerate the anxiety of this ambiguity than to try to escape from it. This is the third way—that of self-exploration rather than running amok or trying to hold on to our previous self-image. By becoming aware of our impulses, we can avoid acting them out or repressing them.

This is a time to explore the unknown and try new ways but stay conscious. We can become aware of our impulses (to move, quit our jobs, leave our lovers) without having to resolve the tension immediately. We can approach these impulses with curiosity rather than suppress them. We can understand even problematic compulsions as full of meaning, inner riches that are getting ready to emerge. Then we can ask ourselves, "What's coming up for me?" instead of fleeing or judging—or acting them out.

In the next chapter we'll look at some ways to get in touch with our "true selves" and discover what really matters.

Relating These Themes to Your Own Experience:

- What have you noticed in terms of your own closure with a youthful identity?
- What's still working for you, and what have you had to let go of?
- Can you identify with any of these types of evasion?
- What would you like to do instead?

Notes

1. Peter Cashorali's *Fairy Tales: Traditional Tales Retold for Gay Men* (HarperSanFrancisco, 1995) includes an engaging story about saying farewell to our golden youth in a gay version of "The Frog Prince."

2. For support in recovery from early abuse, addictions, and homophobia, see *Reclaiming Your Life* by Rik Isensee. Los Angeles: Alyson, 1997.

CHAPTER 4

BEHIND THE MASK

With all the changes we go through at midlife, it's normal to feel uneasy. Aging in the gay community can be experienced as a frightening descent into hell—or as a new adventure (or both)! One reaction is to retreat and try to reclaim one's former self-image as described in "Types of Evasion." But another possibility is to consciously grapple with these emerging forces, moving into the depths, exploring the shadows, reclaiming disowned parts of ourselves, and affirming our true nature.

Rather than simply responding to cues and reinforcements from our parents, society, or even the gay subculture, we become more attuned to the inner resources that are emerging within us. Our sense of self-worth is no longer so vulnerable to outward standards, prizes, awards, or recognition, because we have developed an inner sense of ourselves: "To thine own self be true."

In this chapter we'll explore various ways to get in touch with a more authentic identity.

◆   The Persona   ◆

One of the main reasons for a crisis at midlife is that we have outgrown our previous self-image. Jung calls this early identity the persona, which is like a mask that we show to the world.[1]

It usually tends to be more conventional, conforming to the expectations of our families, friends, and colleagues. Separation from our persona can be equated with death—literally, in the realization that we will die, and figuratively, in the death of our previous self-image.

This is not necessarily a huge crisis for everyone. It generally depends on how in touch we've been with ourselves all along. As mentioned earlier, many of us were forced to confront this mask early on, when we first realized we were gay, and especially when we decided to come out. So we generally have some experience to fall back on as we're coming to terms with this major shift in our self-image—this isn't the first time we've ever had to make a major adjustment in our persona, or how we conceive of ourselves.[2]

Kevin: When I was a boy, I was afraid of being seen as a girl and was even labeled one. I escaped to New York and encountered gay culture there; then my values matured through the AIDS crisis.

I have a great deal of compassion for that younger man—whether it was the kid taunted for being girl-like or for being a faggot. I felt very lost at times, but I got myself out and where I needed to be in order to flourish. Without even realizing it, I did what I needed to do to arrive at a point of adjustment and fulfillment at age 41. With hindsight I can see the logic and necessity of what I did, and I can appreciate what a journey it's been. I'm more extroverted now, thanks to people in my life who made it safe for me to come out. I'm not afraid of being myself any more.

Tony: Growing up gay as an effeminate boy in a macho, Sicilian, working-class neighborhood was incredibly difficult. I didn't have parents who were able to counteract the social messages I was getting—that there was something wrong with me—in fact, they reinforced that message.

I think homophobia had an enormous impact. I grew up with the feeling that I was inferior to the people around me and assumed I'd be unable to achieve wonderful things. It took me many years of being around gay people and seeing what they'd done with their lives before I developed the tools I needed to accomplish my goals.

As I get older and raise my own child, it becomes clearer to me that my childhood was very unhappy and I had no support. Now that I feel good about myself, I'm able to do a lot more than when I was in the throes of depression.

I have a friend who grew up in same area, and she's raising a son there now. He's eight years old, also effeminate, and experiencing a lot of social repercussions, just like I did. But I see how my friend is dealing with it—supporting him to build a good self-concept despite the negative feedback. His experience will be so much better than mine because he has a supportive family. They're acknowledging that sure, you're different, but you have wonderful gifts, and you can put those gifts to work for you; they make you special. That makes all the difference, and I didn't have that.

Randy: I grew up in a black bourgeois family, so they had high expectations for me. I was valedictorian for my high school and had an expansive sense of where I was going. It just seemed to be my destiny to be a role model and a community leader. That was supposed to include finding the right woman and having the cutest, smartest kids.

I went to an elite white school, did well, and became a schoolteacher in the '60s. I was pushed to marry but was honest with myself. It was clear to me that something was missing in that picture, so it didn't make sense to propose marriage. So rather than getting married because it was convenient and expected, I held out.

The Gay Persona

What is a "true self" for gay men? Certainly it has to do with acknowledging we're gay, but it also has to do with affirming our own identity apart from our gay persona as well. Men who think of themselves as gay have transcended the persona of being a straight-identified man. But that often leads to adopting a new persona as being an "out and about" gay man.

This can take many different forms: the in-your-face queer activist, the muscle boy or trendy circuit clubber, the radical fairy, the S/M leatherman, the bear, the A-gay, the dishy queen, or various other personas. These can be developmental reactions to early oppression as well as sincerely thought-out identifications.[3]

Many of us spent years trying to affirm who we were, only to confront a trend toward conformity in the gay subculture—in looks, styles, clothing, and music. Being a slave to fashion is a common phase in adolescence, but by the time we reach midlife, this persona may no longer serve us.

We may try to restore our self-image by finding other ways to fit in, but there's a dawning realization that it's not simply an issue of fitting in and being accepted. There's a loss of interest in the role itself, a search for something more substantial, which is really about getting in touch with our own sense of authenticity. This involves questioning our persona as well as integrating other aspects of our lives.

A more subtle aspect of the gay persona is exemplified by some of the following examples. With many of my clients (as well as colleagues and friends), there has been a tendency to anticipate others' needs—to be the one who is steady and reliable, sensitive and empathic. We were the good boys, the ones who worked very hard, who tried to be there for others. These are certainly wonderful qualities, but for many of us, they came at the expense of not looking out for our own interests.

While being sensitive may simply be a result of temperament, I suspect that such a cooperative persona can also be an attempt to compensate for the fact that we were somehow different. On some level we feared that we would disappoint our family if they ever discovered our true selves, so we developed these endearing qualities to avoid rejection.

Another liability of the "good boy" persona is the fear of being exposed as an impostor. We may be perfectly competent at what we're doing yet still have this sense from early childhood that our secret will be discovered—that we're not quite the idealized boy we pretended to be. This may stem originally from our secret desires, but even when we're out as gay men, this impostor complex can still reverberate through our careers, limit our ability to take care of ourselves, and affect our core sense of self.

Most of us are able to combat this uneasy feeling by looking at our real accomplishments. But at midlife, when everything else is up for grabs, it often reemerges in the form of self-doubt and anxiety. It's tempting to escape from this anxiety through the types of evasion cited earlier. If we can tolerate this uneasiness long enough to explore where it's coming from, then we're more likely to develop a new sense of self that feels solid and in line with our true interests.

Andrew: I was always the responsible one, the one who was reasonable and rational, the peacekeeper. The one who's strong and even-keeled. But what that meant was that I didn't really show my feelings or pay attention to my own needs. My strategy was to be important to others so they would need me, and that made me feel important. I still want to be needed—that's gratifying, but now I want it to be mutual. I want to give to others, and I want something back. I want to be genuine because that's how we can really connect. I'm more revealing and candid now about who I am with my friends and people I work with. I want people to relate to me, not just my persona. If they only relate to my persona, it's hollow. If they fall in love with my mask, it's not with me. The task is really becoming more genuine, both with ourselves and others.

Steve: I was always the good boy and a good student. I was also a "Vulcan" like Mr. Spock—not having to deal with feelings. This was reinforced by medical school, with the professional persona. Now I have less need to please others and more of a desire to please myself.

On the other hand, I've also developed a new persona as an expert, lecturing in my specialty. I find this amusing, like the Wizard of Oz. I realize I'm not the wizard, I'm just the little man behind the curtain. I don't feel like an impostor, more like having fun, playacting, with friends.

Some gay men react against this "good boy" persona by becoming rebels. Healthy rebellion can include standing up for ourselves, social activism, and creative exploration of new modes of dress, sex, and artistic expression. But as mentioned earlier, reactive rebellion can also lead to a devil-may-care attitude, flaming out with drugs, unsafe sex, and other self-destructive behavior.

Professional Personas

A liability for men, especially, is to identify our persona with our profession. Following are a couple of examples of how that can perpetuate an earlier sense of having to prove ourselves.

Hal: The persona I had was one of the food service pro—I could produce this great product cheaper and better than anyone else, and I could do the work of three or four people. Taking care of all the details, being fast and good at projects, knowing how to fix things and make things made me indispensable. People will give up their ability to try or do it because they know I can fix it. I don't do that anymore.

The other one projected onto me is Buddha. I dropped one and killed it off, only to have people trying to put a new one in its place. I try to do things to dissuade that. The opposite of the Buddha is this crass, low-life, unrealized human being who blusters and swears—but that's not working, either. So now I'm going back to just being myself. Others can project what they want, and I'll just have to live with it.

Victor: It doesn't pay to hold on to a tight persona. It was very important to me when I first started out that I was a bona fide licensed psychologist. But I realized I can't hold on to that too tightly. It needs to expand to include other things. I could, I suppose, regrasp or reembrace it, but I don't feel like it. There's no profit in saying, "I'm this and not that." Pretending I'm not things that in fact I am. Am I the grump? Yes. Am I the effusive sparkling presence? Yes. A devoted lover? Yes. A flirt? Yes.

Of course, the persona is not all bad. Sometimes we need to deal with the world in terms of a particular role, like at work, or on a more superficial level. This skillful use of the persona can serve a useful purpose, as Brian indicates:

Brian: I see the persona as being devalued. We see this mask as somehow superficial, but if anything, I've felt the need for a better persona. I've spent plenty of time finding my deeper self, but I've neglected my ability to relate to people at times when it's important not to engage on a deeper level. For example, when cruising, we need a persona, just like a car needs bumpers. Being somewhat superficial at times is not bad.

As gay men, many of us needed to create a persona to pass in the straight world. As a gay subculture, perhaps we tend toward a more superficial persona and hide our deeper self. We've also been creative, playful, and sensual with our gay personas. Maybe we've gotten so good at taking on different roles that there's a danger of getting lost in them, of taking our persona too seriously and neglecting our true selves.

But that doesn't mean the persona is not an important part of one's personality. In some ways I need a better one—maybe with a sense of what to wear, how to chitchat, and how to be relaxed around other gay men.

◆   The Inner Butch and the Inner Fairy   ◆

At midlife aspects of our personalities we've neglected tend to emerge. In Jungian terms, the anima, for men (or the animus, for women) becomes more prominent.[4] The anima is a cluster of characteristics representing our "feminine" side, which some men repress when they are younger. (Gay men may repress their animus, or "masculine" aspects, as well.) As we age and are more secure in our identity, these aspects begin to reappear. Heterosexual men, for example, may become more attuned to relationship issues, more interested in their inner lives, and less competitive with other men. They've already proven themselves and are less vulnerable to judgments about their masculinity. (Whether these aspects are truly "feminine" or are simply relegated to women in our culture, they are commonly left unexplored by most heterosexual men in our culture until later in life.)

Gay men, however, seem less limited by typical masculine constraints.[5] Once we've come out we feel more freedom to explore a wider range of roles. We allow ourselves to play with butch and femme identities. We dress up and parade around with a campy humor that cuts through rigid roles and explodes the usual stereotypes of what it means to be a man or woman in our culture.

As we get older, for many gay men there is a shift, not necessarily as dramatic as for heterosexual men, but nonetheless significant. If we tended to be more masculine-identified, there's often an exploration of receptive roles in sex, emotional connections, and work. Likewise, if we thought of ourselves as effeminate, there may be a shift toward greater assertiveness and

autonomy. The basic idea is that whatever tendencies we neglected when we were younger often reemerge during the second half of life, so we have another chance to delve into these
issues.[6]

This process is similar to coming out, when acknowledging
our sexual orientation challenged our heterosexual self-image.
We confront the persona by getting in touch with our true nature. Confronting the persona then liberates the potential of the
anima, so we can gain access to the neglected parts of our personalities.

It may seem odd to explore the "inner butch" or the "inner
fairy," but there are often gifts awaiting us in these split-off aspects. We may have been repulsed by the harsh masculinity of
our fathers, brothers, or school-yard bullies, for example, and
sworn that we would never be like them. Yet we may end up
throwing out a lot of masculine attributes that have positive sides
as well, such as taking the initiative, thinking clearly, developing
our bodies, or taking risks and competing with other men. By reclaiming these neglected parts, we may be able to expand our
range of behaviors, our attitudes, and even our self-image.

Similarly, we may have identified very strongly with masculine ideals in an effort to protect ourselves. We worked out at
the gym, wore leather, and got butch haircuts, but cut off our
sensitive, artistic sides and hid our emotional vulnerability to
avoid being labeled sissies. Later on, we realize the cost of this
sacrifice was too high: We want to be more expressive emotionally, creatively, and spiritually. So we begin to reclaim the tender
aspects of ourselves we tended to deny earlier on.

Andrew: I claimed the feeling, sensitive part early on, and I
prided myself on developing that. What I'm claiming more
lately is the masculine part of me—owning my power, saying

what I need to say, having the courage to be confrontational or controversial. Those are my current challenges. Expressing my more feminine side is easy for me. To express clearly what I like and what I don't like—that takes courage.

Hal: The anima is my meditative side, the part that can let go and also be receptive to life coming to me. In the past there was a total suppression of her, keeping her at bay. Whenever my family saw that part of me, they tried to kill it, so I put her to sleep. Hiding the need, being tough, making it so I didn't feel. All the work I've done therapeutically has been to reawaken her. She's the one who's intuitive. She tells the male part what to do.

Brian: I've spent a lot of time working with my mother's animus, which I think is one of the main tasks for gay men—working through our mothers' expectations of what we were supposed to be like as a man. I haven't spent as much time yet working with my anima. I think men relate to each other through their animas—by being willing to be vulnerable and by valuing an emotional connection.

Tony: For me, it's trying to be more comfortable with masculine aspects. I grew up being told I was feminine, but I never really accepted it. I tried to hide it, but my self-concept was being an effeminate man. It was a part of myself I hated, because the social repercussions were so bad. I never prayed to be heterosexual, but I remember praying to be more masculine. I had butch guys teach me how to walk and talk. But people always knew I was gay.

I think I'm just coming to terms with this now. There's a part of me that is femme, and that's just who I am. I kind of like it. The guy I'm going out with now treats me in a certain way. It's like I'm a girl and I want to be treated like one, and he does.

I want to be taken care of, but I also want to take care of him.

I don't assume he's stronger than me or more capable than me in any way. At times I'm weak, and I need support and love, and I need to be taken care of. But I have the utmost belief that I can do that for him as well. That's a crucial element in a relationship for me—that I can take care of and respect him and he can do that for me too.

I'm more comfortable now in a masculine role. I can say I'm a "girl" and I want to be treated like one, but I have no illusions about needing someone to take care of me. I'm more flexible going from one role to another. I can be the strong one too, and I feel totally comfortable with that.

Antoine: I guess the masculine side is my animus—I was a priss when I was younger. The only thing that got me by was that I had a brain, and I did my friends' homework. Being smart kept me from getting beat up. But then when I started working out, people assumed I was butch—what a shock!

Steve: I find myself making up for my tendency to isolate by getting engaged in relationships, dealing with feelings, and not being so detached. Now my more neglected part is anger, which gets into shadow stuff. I'm better able to endure things, rather than evading or running away or ignoring.

I feel like I'm changing from introversion to extroversion. I've shifted from reflecting and intrapsychic interests to more public issues. I'm moving from solitary research to more cooperative ventures and sharing more of my findings through public speaking, not just through publishing articles.

Randy: Early on I made a conscious decision to reject traditional male concerns, and that hasn't changed. I was never interested in sports, but because my nephews are into it, I try to stay conversant, but that kind of hypermasculinity never appealed to me, and I had a father who didn't force me. At the same time, I was always afraid of being effeminate. I didn't want to be seen as witty and entertaining but not taken seriously.

Victor: Jung said the first half of life is involved with ego-building, and psychic energy is directed outward, whereas the second half of life is turned inward. There's a sense of change—a fundamental, qualitative shift—a deepening awareness of the spiritual.

When we're younger, we constellate a self by selecting from the vast fund of our experience certain characteristics: This is me—and this is not me. As time goes on, we become more entrenched in that identity. But those parts of ourselves that are less emphasized still remain in the unconscious. At midlife they begin to assert themselves. Those parts of me that I haven't recognized or allowed into consciousness begin to press for acknowledgment.

◆   Only the Shadow Knows   ◆

We've spoken about how the persona is a mask that we present to the world, which protects (and sometimes obscures) our true selves. The anima (or animus) represents those sides of ourselves that we have tended to neglect—the inner butch or the inner fairy. A shy person might get in touch with his dramatic side, for example; or a cynic with his romantic side, an agnostic with his spiritual side, the introvert with his extroversion, and so on.

At midlife we also tend to reencounter whatever aspects of our personalities that we have not only neglected but repressed. The shadow represents aspects of ourselves that we hide from others—at times, even from ourselves—like the inner bitch, the curmudgeon, or the slut.

It's understandable that we would tend to deny aspects of ourselves that seem uncharitable (at best), frightening, or awful—and even humiliating. However, a psychological truth appears to be that acknowledging the shadow makes it less likely to leak out. By getting in touch with our repressed sides, we have more conscious choices about how we want to act in the world. Whereas when the shadow seems too terrible to acknowledge, we try to present a conventional face to the world, but the shadow leaks out, often outside our awareness. Examples include the televangelist who sneaks pornography and abuses his prostitutes, the kindly actress who belittles her children, or the empathic psychotherapist who torments his lover.

This is not just about hypocrisy, because the person may not even be conscious of how he's "leaking" or how he's perceived by others. And because he has repressed this unpleasant side, it's very difficult for him to acknowledge that he's being inconsistent.

However, if we can acknowledge the fact that we have uncharitable feelings at times, that we can be cross and irritable, that we don't always have others' best interests in mind, we have a greater chance of evaluating whether it's a good idea to act on these impulses. We may still decide to do so, but it will be consistent with our conscious will.[7]

Midlife increases our emotional awareness, and our usual defenses break down. The persona collapses, and we release the shadow. One of our tasks is to learn how to tolerate the reemergence of repressed material. We need to find ways to encounter the shadow and grapple with it without simply indulging our impulses, acting out, or running amok. The goal is to integrate these aspects into our personalities, beyond social conventions and roles, in a way that's consistent with our true selves.

Kevin: Growing up, the only part of me that met with positive regard was my academic achievement, and everything else was shadow. Especially my sexuality—and within that my sexual predilections. I felt unmanly, as if I didn't really have a right to be a man. It was helpful for me to discover that I have both masculine and feminine aspects, both of which deserve respect and expression. I give myself permission to express both, and I defend both, and I will do anything possible not to be in a situation where I would have to repress who I am to any appreciable extent. That would be hell. That's where I was in my 20s.

Mario: They say you hate the person who's so much like you. So I try accepting that, and then look for the virtue in that person as I accept more of the virtues in myself.

I used to say whatever I damned well pleased, but now I'm learning to weigh my words, observing what it is I'm saying. I wanted to be in this one relationship so much, but we never even got to know each other. When he was around I was trying too hard to make everything right. I realize now that what I was saying sounded threatening, and he fled. It was my own shadow stuff leaking out, wanting to possess him, but not really paying attention to his needs or what was developing between us.

Hal: I have an incredibly self-destructive bent. Just trying to knock myself off. I'm clear that my shadow tries to kill me all the time. Now I'm more aware of it. Also, I hate rich people, but then that keeps me from having money. All the rich people I happen to know are fucked up. I've got to let this side go so I can have money. I end up sabotaging myself because I equate having money with being a bad person.

Randy: There's a misanthrope in my building—he's particularly vile, always causing problems for others, and every time I ran into this man, I'd feel very angry. A masseur told me because of the tenseness I carried in my shoulders that I had someone under my skin. "You have to let that go."

He explained that I'm letting this man stress me out because he knows he can get this reaction. "You need to understand what it is about him that gets to you. It must be something you fear in yourself."

Generally I get along, feel forgiving. Most people never hear me say I detest someone. He's bigoted, petty, and vindictive. But I had to acknowledge that this person encapsulates my own worst fears.

Tony: I know that whenever I find myself obsessed with someone's shortcomings, that's a sure sign of some aspect of myself that I'm unhappy with. If I start obsessing about a friend, he's so this and so that—I realize now that something's going on with me.

With my son's mother, I would focus on her faults, when in reality what I was really concerned about was my own short-comings as a father. Now I don't do that anymore. When that comes up for me, I realize those intense feelings don't have to do with her; they have to do with me. So I start looking, and I usually find something.

Victor: I'm aware that my shadow is demanding to be ac-knowledged, but because it's unconscious, I have no idea what it looks like until it shows up. Yet I can often tell, after the fact, that I've integrated these shadow aspects.

For example, I have a much better time dancing now than I did five years ago, because I accept that I'm a flirt. I used to have a lot of judgments about people who flirted. I used to think they were bad, they shouldn't be doing that, it can hurt people or lead people on. But I realized it's harmless, and anyone seeing me would know it's harmless. Now I can see flirtatious people and smile rather than feel enraged, because I accept that part of myself. It doesn't have to be a contradiction—I can be a devoted lover as well as a flirt. I like it.

The shadow contains repressed material—but not all repressed material is "bad"—it simply wasn't acceptable to think of ourselves that way, so we pushed it aside. For gay men, sometimes feeling good about ourselves, being proud of our accomplishments, or recognizing our capabilities is relegated to the shadow, because it doesn't seem OK to acknowledge those aspects of ourselves.

Brian: There can be positive aspects in the shadow too. I'm working on the fact that some of my self-confidence and self-esteem are in my shadow. The shadow is not just dark and bad. But it often contains things you've decided are bad for you—that you've disowned or split off. In my family, my sister was self-asserting, but I saw how badly that went over with my parents, so I adopted an adaptive, compliant personality, putting self-assertion in my shadow. I was also influenced by feminism and had a tendency to split off any sense of power or self-confidence and relegate it to the shadow because in the larger society male power seemed like a bad thing. Now I'm trying to reclaim these qualities for myself.

The other aspect of the shadow is that it often represents an early awareness of the "divine," or the dissolution of the ego. It's split off not because it's bad, but because it seems overpowering, as the following example illustrates.

Andrew: I see a force in me that is so huge, if I yield and surrender to it, I feel annihilated. That's scary—but it's a merging of my ego into the infinite. It started out in dreams, as a force that was so powerful I would get squashed. Terror and awe, like Moses with the burning bush, or an ant in the face of a tornado—totally at the whim of that force. To face that has taken huge amounts of courage, to stand in the face of internal annihilation—that I could dissolve and face the disappearance of my existence. That's death, right there.

As gay boys many of us felt the need to cut off our inner resources in order to survive. We hid the inner fairy, the creative, intuitive, sensitive, and open parts of ourselves so that we wouldn't be humiliated, tormented, or killed. Some of us became overly adaptive and hid our self-assertion; others rebelled in ways that were self-defeating. We survived as best we could, finally affirming our true nature as gay men. As adults we can grieve for our losses, but there is also a fountain of healing and rebirth within the despair and suffering. By reclaiming these aspects of ourselves, we can enrich our lives and reach out to others to share this bounty.

Relating These Themes to Your Own Experience

- What was your persona as you were growing up, before you came out?
- What was your "gay persona" after coming out?
- How has that changed over time?
- What aspects of your personality, whether masculine or

feminine, introverted or extroverted, are now beginning to reemerge?

• What "shadow" aspects about yourself that you tended to deny in the past can you now accept or deal with more successfully?

Notes

1. Carl Jung: "The term *persona* is really a very appropriate expression for this, for originally it meant the mask once worn by actors to indicate the role they played.... Fundamentally, the persona is nothing real; it is a compromise between individual and society as to what a man should appear to be..." Cited in *Persona* by Robert Hopcke, p. 13. Boston: Shambhala, 1995. Hopcke also addresses the impact of being "social outsiders" on gay persona development, pp. 121-146.

2. Some research indicates that coping successfully with coming out creates a "crisis competence," which increases our ability to resolve other conflicts later in life. "Adult Development and Aging: A Gay Perspective" by D.C. Kimmel. *Journal of Social Issues,* 34 (3), pp. 113-130, 1978.

3. The whole controversy over "queer" versus "gay" identity reminded me of a similar discussion among radical groups during the '70s: "homosexuals" were seen as still in the closet, "gays" as focused only on gay liberation and assimilation, whereas the word "faggot" was reclaimed to represent the "vanguard of the anti-imperialist struggle."

4. "The anima...functions as the medium between the ego and the unconscious, as does the persona between the ego

and the environment." Carl Jung, cited in Hopcke, p. 23.

5. "Sex Role Endorsement Among Homosexual Men Across the Life Span," by B.E. Robinson, P. Skeen, and C. Flake-Hobson. *Archives of Sexual Behavior* 11:355-359, 1982. (Cited by Robert Kertzner in *Textbook of Homosexuality and Mental Health*; see note 11, Chapter 10.)

6. In *The Seasons of a Man's Life,* Levinson describes a number of dualities that we are dealing with at middle age: young/old, destruction/creation, attachment/separateness, and masculine/feminine. See note 1, Chapter 2.

7. See *Owning Your Own Shadow: Understanding the Dark Side of the Psyche* by Robert A. Johnson. San Francisco: HarperSanFrancisco, 1991.

CHAPTER 5

PHYSICAL AND SEXUAL CHANGES

At midlife we gradually become more aware of physical changes: weight gain and wrinkles, gray hair, and changes in vision—but also how our bodies don't seem to bounce back as quickly after intense exertion or overindulgence.

Even though these initial shifts in our appearance and stamina are often quite subtle, they can have a severe emotional impact when they're recognized as signs of inevitable decline—and mortality. They can also serve as a wake-up call for men who have not really taken care of themselves or paid particular attention to their bodies. Many gay men at midlife embark on a more healthful diet and exercise regimen, not only to stay healthy, but to maintain their looks and physique. In this chapter, we'll take a look at common physical and sexual changes, how to take care of ourselves physically, and expand our notions of what it means to be gay and attractive at midlife.

◆   Changes in Body Image   ◆

There is a lot that we can do to stay fit and healthy. At the same time, it's also better not to overdo it, so we don't hurt ourselves physically and then give up altogether. Many men feel intimidated by the whole gym culture, which seems to accentuate youthful, hunky bodies as the ultimate ideal for gay men. We can exercise to keep fit and not judge our bodies with unrealistic comparisons to men who are half our age.

As Tony became more accepting of himself and his body, this transformed his experience of working out. Instead of comparing himself with others, he was able to concentrate on taking care of himself. This allowed him to interact with other men in a more natural way.

Tony: The gym has always been intimidating to me. I used to walk in with this apprehension that I was somehow less than others. I've carried a lot of shame with me my whole life, and only recently am I learning how to shed that cloak of shame. My whole experience at the gym is different now. Going to the gym builds my self-esteem instead of taking away from it. Now I can walk into the gym with the thought that I have just as much right to be there as anyone else. I can feel proud of myself and perceive myself as a desirable and attractive man. Because I'm feeling more confident, my interactions flow in a more natural way—like one equal talking to another—instead of feeling "less than" and needing to prove that I'm not.

Not all gay men have a burning desire to keep up with the current "body culture" at the gym. In the next example Kevin discloses how physical changes have affected his self-esteem.

Insofar as our self-worth is dependent upon physical attractiveness, we're likely to feel worse as our looks inevitably fade. If we haven't done so already, at midlife we need to develop other sources of feeling good about ourselves, as Kevin describes.

Kevin: This is painful to say, but midlife has involved letting go of viewing myself as physically attractive. I had a lover die of AIDS, and after that I gained weight that I've never lost. That forced home the implications of being less physically appealing than I used to be. It's a loss of social power and a loss of self-esteem.

I don't like the changes in my body, and it's difficult not to compare myself to images that appear in the media. I feel alienated from the youth culture in bars and dance clubs. I'm not a part of the visible Castro scene, and when I go there I can end up feeling devalued—even scorned.

But striving to keep up with younger men or the current body culture just isn't worth it to me. I have other interests and friends that I choose to spend my time on. There are enough other areas aside from physical attractiveness to compensate for the loss of self-esteem. I love my friends, my relationship, profession, and other interests, such as classical music. The older I get, the more meaning great works of music have for me. It was impossible in my 20s to appreciate the depth of music that I enjoy now.

Similarly, I don't appreciate taking drugs and staying up all night anymore. I suppose there's appropriate behavior at each stage in life. I feel fairly well-adjusted to midlife, but it's an ongoing process. So long as someone I find attractive finds me attractive and enjoys my body, I won't really suffer in a meaningful way. And I enjoy sex with men my age.

Physical Changes

Following is an overview of common physical changes, with some comments describing how other men have been dealing with them.

The loss of collagen in our skin gradually leads to wrinkles and sagging. Sunlight contributes greatly to aging the skin. Sunburn is the worst, but even tanning (in the sun as well as tanning booths) can lead to early collagen loss and premature wrinkles. New laser surgeries can smooth out the skin and eliminate the fat under puffy eyes. On the other hand, laugh lines and crow's feet are inevitable and give character to your face. If you like a little color, some of the new sunless tanning creams look pretty natural and don't damage your skin.

Mario: I like the aging process, the way the face changes. I feel good about the lines in my face. I see older women with their faces stretched back by plastic surgery, and it looks so artificial. The people I'm attracted to are those who have character faces. My face has sharp features, nice skin, but I love my friend Ernie, who has a big broken nose and lines forming on his face. I can see how he'll look at 50 or 60, and that's great. I find that visually appealing and a sign of character.

Brian: Fifty isn't as old as it used to be. Apart from HIV, we're staying healthier longer and living longer, and maybe our culture will support us growing older in a different way. Advertising has to reflect the aging boomers by talking about "well-earned wrinkles" and "different types of beauty."

So much advertising is oriented toward preventing, reversing, and disguising the loss of hair, you would think it was a national obsession or a major source of shame. The fact is that most men turn gray and experience some degree of hair loss over the course of their lives. Like many other physical changes at midlife, it takes some adjustment. Thinning and graying hair can affect our self-image and how we imagine other people perceive us.

Male pattern baldness can be temporarily reversed with medication in some men, but it returns as soon as the medication is stopped. Some improvement has been made in hair transplant surgery, but it's crucial to evaluate the results of other customers. Hairpieces look more natural than they used to. Lots of men use rinses to cover the gray and feel good about looking as youthful as they feel.

The other side of this quandary is that many men look great without their hair! Accepting gray hair and natural hair loss can liberate us from self-judgment and free us from anticipated rejection. Luckily, even within the gay community there is more appreciation and even a greater attraction for men with various degrees of hair loss and gray hair. This may be a result of the natural aging of our population, as well as a shift toward more masculine fashions and hairstyles.

Mario: Gray hair's a bummer. I have a full head of salt-and-pepper hair. For a while I was just letting it get gray—I looked like Norman Bates's mother. So I started doing a hair rinse. I don't feel old, but my hair would certainly give it away. Also with my line of work, as a performer, salt-and-pepper doesn't look that good—when it's all white, I'll let it go. I'll look like some ancient Montezuma god.

Changes in vision, body aches and pains that don't go away as quickly as they used to, and weight gain are also common complaints at midlife.

Randy: My hair is not naturally this color; I've got a lot of gray.

My visual acuity is going. I can't read a map in the car anymore. But basically I've been lucky around health. I recently visited with some 30-year-old relatives who said I was hard to keep up with.

Antoine: My eyes are getting bad. I have to exercise harder to keep in shape. My memory isn't as good as it was. Now I have to think a little about what I was going to do. I can't eat some of the same things I used to.

I have holes in my retina, due partly to aging, and partly heredity. Some of the debris has landed in certain spots, which clouds my vision. All someone needs to do is punch me in the head, and my right eye will go blind. I don't want all this eye stuff to be happening to me. I want to do things, experience life before my eyes get worse.

Handling changes seems easier, because I accept them more; I don't fight them as much, especially this eye problem—you learn to live with it; otherwise I'd just hang around the house and mope. I see a doctor every week to monitor it. I have three doctors taking care of me—it's wonderful attention.

Andrew: My body aches more in general. I have an increasing awareness of the vulnerability of my body—something could go wrong, and I could die. My hair's turning gray, and it's harder to lose weight. I'm not freaked about it—weight gain has been a lifelong issue. Now it's even harder to keep my weight down, so that's distressing.

Natural Body Types

Every body is unique, but most of us fit into one of three general body types: ectomorphs, or slender guys; endomorphs, or husky guys; and mesomorphs, or muscular guys. Our current culture idolizes the mesomorphs, those naturally muscular guys who build up muscle easily. Instead of simply accepting our natural body types, stocky guys often wish they were skinnier, the skinny guys wish they had more muscles, and the muscular guys—well, they always think they should be bigger! What's a guy to do?

While it's true that some slender guys can become more defined if they work hard enough, it's absurd for them to compare themselves with guys who have a muscular build to begin with. And husky guys can be in great shape and plenty strong and still be big rather than thin.

Steroids

Steroid use has gone way up among gymgoers in the gay community. These drugs have long been present in body-building culture, but their recent surge in popularity is probably due to their use among HIV-positive men to build muscle mass and ward off wasting syndrome. Their friends have noticed how hunky they look, and steroid use has spread throughout gay gyms across the country.[1]

Some men figure, What harm can it do? They love the big, sculpted look steroids provide that no amount of bodybuilding seemed to give them otherwise. So a new norm of a rock-hard, steroid-induced physical type has arisen, and many men feel they need to live up to it. This can be pretty depressing, especially for men at midlife who assume this is a new standard we should aspire to instead of just trying to stay fit.

There are some real dangers in steroid abuse. It interrupts your testosterone production and shrinks your testicles. It can lead to acne and more serious problems, such as liver and kidney damage. And, strangely, steroid use sometimes leads to breast enlargement, because the steroids can convert to estrogen, the female hormone.[2]

Steroid abuse can also contribute to "'roid rages"—out-of-control reactions to normal stresses and disappointments, which can destroy relationships and get you into lots of trouble. The literature records major mood disorders—ranging from irritability to mania and bouts of depression as well as increased aggression, delusions, and paranoia.[3]

The relatively small doses prescribed for men who have low testosterone levels are reported to cause increased irritability but not the larger mood swings associated with steroid abuse.[4] Everyone starts out thinking he'll be able to moderate his use. But it's easy to fall into a bodybuilding culture that distorts your body image so that you're never satisfied—you always think you should be bigger and more sculpted, until you end up looking like the staggering hulks you see lumbering around the gym.[5]

We don't have to buy into these exaggerated and distorted notions of what makes a "perfect body." If you look at erotic magazines or even popular films from the '40s through the '70s, you can see there was a wider variety of male physical types that were considered attractive. We weren't limited to smooth muscle boys.

Rather than comparing ourselves to others or aspiring to an ideal that's only attainable by 1% of the population, it's better to accept our basic physique. We can exercise to keep fit and look our best without using steroids to fulfill some hypermasculine fantasy.

Mario: I find myself striving less, not trying to meet others' expectations. I go to the gym when I want, to make myself feel better, not to get some Greek body for others.

That competitiveness isn't there.

Tony: The honest truth is, I feel I'm more desirable now because I'm more grounded. Physically, I look fine, that's not a big issue. My looks are fading, but that doesn't really concern me. I think 45- to 50-year-old men can look great. I see it all the time. Even though I joke about it, I don't feel like an old queen who's fading into some vast wasteland.

Staying in Shape

Fat on men tends to accumulate around the middle, with a potbelly and love handles. Even for men who run regularly, it takes increasingly more distance to maintain the same weight as they grow older—especially if they continue to consume the same number of calories!

After 35 the body also loses lean muscle mass. But this can be reversed to a great extent if we exercise. So in addition to aerobic exercise to keep the heart healthy and to avoid the accumulation of fat, it's also helpful to include some strength-building exercise to keep up your muscle mass. An added benefit is that muscles stimulated by exercise continue to metabolize fat even after you've stopped exercising.

Dieting versus Exercise

Numerous studies demonstrate that "dieting" doesn't work—if by dieting we mean a severe deprivation of calories over a short period of time for the purpose of losing a substantial amount of weight. The reason that rapid weight loss is difficult to sustain is that you lose as much lean body mass as fat. Then when you go off the diet, you often feel so deprived that you put the weight right back on, but this time it's mostly fat![6]

Of course it makes sense to pay attention to what you eat, and it's possible to change how you eat so you can maintain a more healthful diet over time, rather than getting caught up in a cycle of severe deprivation and overindulgence. A low-fat diet of whole grains, plenty of fruits and vegetables, and moderate amounts of protein can help you feel good and stay in shape.

It's also nearly impossible to lose weight without starving yourself if you're not exercising. Even a light amount of exercise, such as a brisk walk, is far better than none at all. Some form of aerobic exercise for 20 minutes three times a week is helpful, not only for your heart and your physique, but also for your mental balance. This is due to the release of endorphins during aerobic exercise, which can elevate your mood and help you feel better about yourself in general.

Victor: Aging has made my body less tolerant of not taking care of it. If I want to maintain my weight, I have to exercise and be more conscious now of what I eat. If I skip only a few days, my body changes more quickly, and it takes longer to get back to where I was. In the past, if I went on a trip, I didn't worry about exercising. Now I make sure I have a place to work out. No one would notice but me, but I'd feel flabbier and more lethargic.

Brian: I have the body of a midlife person—I'm certainly not 30 anymore—but inside I feel stronger and better. I notice wrinkles in my face, my hair's thinning and turning gray, but I'm actually in better shape now than I was 15 years ago. When I was in a relationship, I let my body go. Now I'm 50 and single and I'm trying to stay healthy. I recently lost 15 pounds through aerobic exercise.

◆ Daddies and Masters and Bears (Oh, My!) ◆

Taking on certain roles seems to be one way that some older men have connected with younger guys (and also with each other). Daddies and masters frequently incorporate fantasy and role-play into their sexual contacts. Whether this can be sustained beyond a particular scene depends on the willingness of both partners to communicate what else they want—and also to see the person behind the role. The bear scene has created an alternative to smooth young muscle boys, in which husky, hairy guys can celebrate their own physical types and validate their attractions.

Some men are not interested in roles. They don't see themselves as masters or daddies or bears, and they resist being put into those positions by partners who may have a hard time seeing them as anything but a particular role in their fantasy. Younger men encounter this problem, too—they're often objectified as twinks or hunks. And some men with large endowments complain that they're often seen only in terms of stud fantasies, rather than being appreciated for who they are as real human beings with their own personalities and desires.

Of course, we can play around with different roles without getting caught up in them or thinking that's all there is. Perhaps midlife offers an opportunity to make more conscious choices—we can engage in the role in a playful way but not feel compelled to stay there, and we can also drop the role and engage with our true selves.

Racial Attractions

Some men have dealt with similar issues regarding cross-cultural and interracial dating. They may be attracted to a particular race or cultural group, yet be surprised when their boyfriend doesn't fit the expected stereotype. Many men of color want to be seen as themselves, and not objectified as a black stud or an exotic, submissive Asian or a passionate Latino.

At the same time some men of color who enjoy interracial dating don't want to be accused of internalized racism just because they have a Euro-American boyfriend. As a community, it would probably help us to address issues around desire, objectification, and cultural differences surrounding race, ethnicity, class, and age. At midlife perhaps we're at a better place to engage in these discussions by listening to one another's experience, rather than trying to establish a "correct" line or policy for everyone.

Randy: As an African-American, it seems to me that our community hasn't addressed its own racism. The gay community projects itself as being accepting, but most black people don't feel as though we've been accepted.

The gay community has been a disappointment to me because it hasn't been any less racist than the larger society. It's always some white middle-class male who's sought out as a spokesperson, with the arrogance of his own narrow experience as though he's speaking for everyone. With the standards of beauty depicted in the gay media, the clubbiness of social events, I usually feel on the edge of a white gay male world rather than part of it.

When gay men make analogies between the gay experience and the civil rights movement, black people often feel they're riding on our coattails without having earned that right. If the gay community were more willing to address its own racism, that would go a long way toward finding common goals in our struggles.

◆ Changes in Sexuality ◆

There are a number of changes that take place in men's sexuality as we age. In a sexually oriented culture, these changes can be disturbing. It's helpful to recognize expectable changes so you don't assume something is fundamentally wrong with you.[7]

- Spontaneous erections are less frequent.
- Erections arise less often in response to visual cues or fantasies.
- As a consequence, we often require more physical stimulation to get hard and to stay hard.
- It takes longer to get an erection.
- Erections are generally less firm and don't stay hard as long.
- It takes longer to come.
- Ejaculations are less forceful, and we ejaculate less semen.
- The refractory period is longer—after ejaculating, it takes more time to become aroused again than when we were younger.

- At midlife some circumcised men report less sensation in the glans (head) of their penis.[8]

Enlarged Prostate

In midlife many men develop an enlarged prostate, which can constrict the urethra, causing more frequent, less forceful urination. You may have to get up more frequently at night to urinate. It often takes more effort to shake out the last drops of urine. If some remains in the urethra, it can be forced out when we bend over by compressing the prostate. This is annoying but usually harmless unless the urethra becomes too constricted. After age 40 it's a good idea to have your prostate checked.

Impotence

Lack of an erection is a common complaint at midlife. It's helpful to have a urological exam to see whether anything is wrong physically. If you normally get erections when you masturbate and when you sleep, there's a good chance that nothing's wrong with the "plumbing."

Certain medications, such as antidepressants, can contribute to delayed ejaculation or lack of sexual desire. Diabetes and surgery for prostate cancer can also lead to impotence. There are a number of temporary treatments available now for physically based impotence, including shots and oral medications.

There can be many other reasons for not getting an erection, such as drinking too much, being tired, or just not being very interested. Being annoyed or distracted by work, having unresolved conflicts with your partner, feeling depressed, or being concerned about sexual safety can also contribute to momentary impotence.

Performance anxiety is probably the most frustrating cause of erectile failure that isn't physiologically based. This is because we're concentrating so much on whether we're getting hard rather than paying attention to the erotic sensations that would normally lead to an erection. If you felt disappointed or humiliated by a previous erectile failure or rejection, this can lead to associating sex with anxiety. While there are some men who find anxiety a turn-on, for most men it's definitely not the greatest aphrodisiac. What could have been an isolated incident ends up perpetuating itself—you feel anxious about whether you'll be able to perform the next time, and that anxiety actually inhibits your erection.

It's helpful to take the pressure off a particular encounter by simply deciding that it doesn't matter whether you get an erection or not. Giving each other a massage can help you relax, and messing around in other ways can be a lot of fun. Paradoxically, deciding beforehand that you're not going to have anal sex can lead to getting an erection after all!

Some men complain that the problem is not getting the erection; it's keeping it up. First you get hard, then you pull out a condom and slip it on, then you have to get back into position. You can use up so much energy with these acrobatics that your body decides it needs more blood in your muscles, then blip! there goes your erection. Sometimes it's helpful for the "top" to be on the bottom. Try lying on your back and letting your partner get you hard. Then he can ease himself onto you.

As we age there's often a release from the sexual urgency of youth, which many men find a great relief. They realize that erotic feelings are not limited to the genitals. With less emphasis on performance and ejaculation, some gay men report an increase in sexual pleasure.[9] Some men have experimented with breathing exercises and genital stimulation to expand pleasurable sensations throughout the body. With ejaculation no longer the end goal, they describe these sensations as "multiple orgasms."

Brian: I find that I have more desire for cuddling, intimacy, touch, and massage than for orgasms. Of course, that might be different if I had a boyfriend.

Antoine: I'm not as horny as I used to be, although my partner's sex drive is as strong as it's ever been, even though he's nearly 20 years older.

Steve: I find myself looking more—anyone in his 30s looks cute now. I never felt like part of the gay scene at clubs, so the shift to the periphery wasn't a big deal. It no longer feels necessary to be in the game. I'm finding a shift from lust to friendship, like heterosexual lust moves more to family concerns. I'm trying to be aware of the journey and not give up on finding someone or stopping too early—like the guy who gave up finding a boyfriend and got a dog instead.

Randy: Mostly I'm aware of the absence of a sex life, and that's been going on for years. I'm too picky, yet I keep falling for the wrong orientation—either straight or unavailable. Not much change physically, although I guess I'm not as fixated on sex as a healthy 20-year-old would be, but I didn't realize I was gay until I was 30 anyway. At midlife I'm less sexually active than when I first came out.

Victor: Occasionally it's been distressing that I'm not as sexually charged as I used to be. But it's a relief more than anything because that energy used to run me. Now it's more of an ally instead of this wild beast that I need to tame.

Andrew: I don't feel much of a lessening in frequency or desire. Erections are softer, and it takes longer to get really hard. I feel some distress in trying to fit into the gay culture—most personal ads cut off at 45, so I feel less desirable. I know that's not true, because some men are attracted to older men. But since I like younger guys, I feel like my options are limited.

Kevin: I noticed my refractory time is greater—in my 20s within minutes I could come again. But I seldom think about that, and I don't feel limited. I have much less promiscuous sex and much less interest in sex for its own sake. Yet at the same time, I feel much more sex-positive and more accepting of my own sexuality. Life is short, so why not enjoy what you like. I'm not ashamed of my sexuality, and I don't have to drink or do drugs to enjoy it.

My idea of what sex is has broadened. When I was young, it was meeting someone and having hot sex immediately. There wasn't much of a repertoire or breadth. Now just looking at someone beautiful or attractive can be a complete experience. I don't have to consummate it with a sex act. Flirting is fun, but it doesn't have to go anywhere. Affection and physical closeness in general are vastly more important to me than "hot" sex, which I still enjoy on occasion—but I'd never trade it for the fulfillment of my partner's company. Overall, sex is just less important.

Strangely, the fact that sex is less important relieves me of a burden. Because it's not the center of my life, that frees me to partake in the rest of the world. There are many pleasures, important satisfactions and issues beyond my own self-pleasuring that are worthwhile getting involved with. I think a preoccupation with sex got in the way of that for me.

In the next chapter we'll look at the impact of these sexual changes on dating and connecting with other guys.

Relating These Themes to Your Own Experience:

- What changes have you noticed in your own body?
- How would you like to take care of yourself physically?
- How has your sexual functioning changed over time?
- What have these changes meant to you?

Notes

1. See *Life Outside* by Michelangelo Signorile, p. 140. New York: HarperCollins, 1997.
2. Ibid., p. 163.
3. Ibid., p. 165-66. (From a citation in the *Journal of the American Medical Association,* 1994.)
4. Ibid., p. 165.
5. Harrison G. Pope Jr. is a psychiatrist who describes "muscle dysmorphics" as men who have a "pathological preoccupation with their degree of muscularity." Cited in *Scientific American,* March 1998, p. 24.
6. See *Smart Exercise: Burning Fat, Getting Fit* by Covert Bailey. Boston: Houghton Mifflin, 1994. *Fit Over Forty* by James Rippe. New York: William Morrow, 1996. *Men's Fitness Magazine's Complete Guide to Health and Well-Being* with Kevin Cobb. New York: HarperCollins, 1996.

7. See *Male Sexuality* by Bernie Zilbergeld, p. 332. New York: Bantam, 1981.

8. *The Joy of Uncircumcising!* by Jim Bigelow. Aptos, Calif: Hourglass, 1995.

9. "Life-History Interviews of Aging Gay Men," by D.C. Kimmel. *International Journal of Aging and Human Development,* 10, 239-248, 1979.

CHAPTER 6

SEX AND THE SINGLE GAY GUY

So much advertising, commerce, and money in the gay community seems to be oriented toward sex. Sex attracts our attention; sex beguiles and distracts us. Being aroused by other men is how many of us realized we were gay, and sexual liberation formed a cornerstone of gay liberation. Images of sex between men permeate our subculture. Sex sells. The impression we often get from many gay publications is "the more sex, the better."

At midlife many gay men begin to question the importance of sex in our lives. This is due in part to the natural physiological changes mentioned previously, so that there isn't quite the same urgency in our sexual appetite. But I believe it's also due to an increased level of self-acceptance, so we're not as compelled to seek out sex as a form of self-validation. In this chapter we'll take a look at how these changes affect our desires for dating and finding a relationship.

◆ Sex and Dating at Midlife ◆

By the time we reach midlife, we often feel less driven by sexual urges. Many of us want more of a connection, not just to get off. A sense of closeness can be greatly enhanced by sharing what we're feeling and saying what we really want from each other. The willingness to communicate feelings of vulnerability can deepen our experience of emotional intimacy.

For some men, what worked previously in terms of quick sexual contact is no longer satisfying. But it takes a while to figure out what else to do. And it also takes some effort to find other men who are on the same wavelength, who are willing to communicate about what they want—not only sexually but in terms of relating to each other as real human beings.

Mario: I find it easy to pick up men to have sex. I think that's a result of the time when I came out—we didn't shake hands, we shook dicks. But what I'm realizing is that a pickup is not a relationship and that it's not necessarily a good way to get to know someone. So I'm having to reevaluate all that. Do I want to have sex right away or get to know him first? Even if he's cute, he may be a horrible person. Yet it's exciting to get to know someone.

Being a Pisces, I tend to fall in love too easily and get my heart broken. I'm still vulnerable to those ups and downs. To be rejected in general is painful. I have the clarity to see what's coming, but I'll have fun anyway and pay the consequences, whether it's a hangover or a broken heart. I may hurt from it, but it doesn't stop me from taking chances. If it backfires, tough. So I'll sulk and then move on.

There has been a lot of press in recent years about settling down, especially in response to the AIDS crisis and in light of the movement to legalize same-sex marriage.[1] Some men perceive an emphasis on monogamy as the result of a "sex panic" that blames recreational sex for the spread of AIDS.[2] The debate is often framed as a struggle of "assimilationists" versus "sex radicals," but the right to marry and the right to sexual self-determination are not mutually exclusive. Gay men enjoy a wide range of sexual interests: Some men want to get married, some prefer recreational sex—and some men are exploring both!

It's clear from the debate over this issue that there are still plenty of men who enjoy sexual abandon. Recreational sex can also be conscious and safe. Many men are exploring erotic massage, leather, and tantric sex as paths of healing the split between sex and spirituality, while others revel in momentary sexual contact in a primal, tribal way.[3] Sex can be used to feel good, to soothe ourselves, to connect with others, or to shore up our self-esteem. There's nothing wrong with sex, even for its own sake, but for some men recreational sex can mask their longing for emotional intimacy as well.

In many sexual venues, such as bars, baths, and dance clubs, there seems to be an unspoken expectation that we'll have hot sex but not talk about what's going on. The problem with these unspoken norms is that it feels risky even to acknowledge them, much less suggest any alternative. I've seen men in my practice who feel uncomfortable with fast-paced sexual contact, but they hesitate to bring it up for fear of rejection. Wanting to slow things down or talk about their expectations doesn't mean they're "sex-negative." They simply want to expand their repertoire of sexual involvements to include emotional intimacy.

I realize that men who feel satisfied with recreational sex are not as likely to seek therapy about it, so I may be seeing a self-selected sample. For some gay men, however, the emotional bond is the neglected part. Sex is the lure, but if that's all they ever get, they miss having a deeper connection.

Although coming out forced us to grapple with a major shift in our self-concept, for many of us there is still a mistrust of other men that can interfere with emotional connections. A relationship often elicits our own unresolved issues around abandonment and homophobia. By talking about what's coming up for us rather than fleeing, we have the opportunity to resolve these issues and expand our capacity for intimacy. Part of this authentic connection is not only with another man but with ourselves. We realize what's really important to us, and we're willing to speak up about it and engage with other men about our thoughts, feelings, and values.

So how can we indulge our fantasies, be playful and sexual, while still treating one another with respect and caring? The key lies in communicating our feelings and expectations. Roles and fantasies can be fun and stimulating, like an appetizer. In a particular scene, maybe that's all you're interested in. But other delights may await us if we stick around for the main course—to connect with our hearts and minds as well as sexually.

Mario: I thought being gay was having sex with lots of people, but I've realized that isn't very satisfying. I had a sense of fulfillment with David [who died three years ago]. I realize now I don't know how to date, and I'm not sure I want to spend the energy. Listening to a lot of younger gay men, who are looking for a gay marriage, I'm not sure they want to make that commitment. They say they want what I want, but they don't have the tools or energy to make it happen. In reality it's a lot of hard work.

In the following example Tony talks about reentering the dating scene at midlife after his lover died from AIDS. He also describes struggling with his attraction to anonymous sex—how in some ways it's not that satisfying, yet it still has a certain allure. During times of stress, when looking for sex seems most appealing, he'd like to do more nurturing things for himself. Recently he started to date someone, but he's questioning whether they're sexually compatible. Should he continue this relationship and just get his sexual needs met elsewhere? Or would that just lead him back into more anonymous sex?

Tony: My lover of 14 years died four years ago. I went through a long period of mourning, not dating and not wanting to. The last time I dated was in my mid 20s, during the '70s. Now I'm 43, and it's a whole different scene. As I date men and get involved emotionally and sexually, sex sometimes loses its appeal.

I'm still struggling with sexuality. I've often been hypersexual, especially if I'm feeling down or confused and overwhelmed. My initial impulse is to go out and have sex—but I only feel worse, even if I felt better at the moment. I'm still attracted to anonymous sex, and at times I feel compelled to participate, whether it's in the locker room, a bookstore, the park, or the baths.

I don't do it as much as I used to, but the desire is still there. As a young man, I figured when I met Mr. Right, this would stop naturally. When I was in my 20s, I saw men in their 40s and hoped I wouldn't be like them, still coming to the bookstore or bushes to get laid when I'm in my 40s. But as I get older, I realize this could go on. I see men in their 60s still cruising the parks.

I've learned what I can do for myself that's nurturing and sustaining—and what isn't. Anonymous sex might make me feel better for the moment, but I know if I do it I'll just spiral downward. If I do something more nurturing, like meditating, reading, or if I go out with a friend, take a walk in the park, that can help me through a bad period. It's taken me a long time to learn that.

I could imagine settling down with my current boyfriend, who I find emotionally compatible. I like being with someone my own age; he's good with my nine-year-old son; we like doing a lot of the same things, like traveling and going out, but I'm not that sexually attracted. We sleep together and cuddle in bed, but sex isn't great.

We could live together and provide each other with emotional support, and I could still get sex somewhere else. He also enjoys anonymous sex; he goes to blow buddies once a week, so maybe that's how it's going to be. But having that kind of relationship doesn't really appeal to me.

With my lover who died, sex was charged and passionate and incredible for a couple of years, and yes, that faded over time, but not completely until the end. Even when he was skinny and sick, literally a shadow of the guy he'd been, I still found him sexy—his curly hair, his dick, just the way he walked and smiled at me was sexy.

◆ Countering Shame About Being Single ◆

Many guys at midlife approach the whole dating scene with a sense of dread. If they've been out of circulation for a while, it can seem rather intimidating, especially at dance clubs where most of the men appear to be in their 20s to early 30s. Some men go about their business, getting together with friends or pursuing other interests, figuring they'll run across someone in the course of their normal routine. But years go by, they become more set in their ways, and it becomes increasingly obvious that they're not meeting anyone.

Heterosexual men are often gratified by having women in their lives who look after their practical and emotional needs, whereas gay men often develop both a practical and emotional self-sufficiency. It takes effort to pursue other interests. We wonder if we're too set in our ways, and it's hard to imagine being able to live with anyone else. It just seems like too much trouble.

Shame about being single has been a common theme in my support group. We've internalized the notion that it's somehow better to be in a relationship, so there must be something essentially wrong with us if we've arrived at midlife and we're still single (or no longer in a relationship). What's this about?

Part of it has to do with wanting very much to have that special connection with another man, and feeling sad at times for not having it, and we begin to wonder whether we ever will. A common fear of gay men at midlife is that if we haven't made that connection by the time we're middle-aged, it's too late. We may assume that our youthful attractiveness is gone and that we can't compete in the gay meat market. Being single at midlife, it's easy to feel as though we've somehow missed the boat.

Yet many gay men at midlife feel that they simply weren't ready for a serious relationship when they were younger. Perhaps we have a developmental time line that's different from heterosexual coupling. Maybe it's also a reflection of the times when many of us came out—the emphasis was on sexual liberation rather than finding a relationship. Some men may be more in touch with their desire for intimate contact because of the losses they've experienced through AIDS.

In the next two examples, Brian and Randy describe how at age 50 it's easy to internalize the message that something's wrong with us if we're still single at midlife—and how they've tried to deal with it.

Brian: I've had this limiting belief that you can only fall in love in your 20s and 30s. You become attached and live out the rest of your life together. That's the romantic ideal that few people actually experience, and it keeps me from being open to other possibilities. I feel sad about not being with someone where we could look back at being 25 together. That's simply not going to happen.

At 40 I was in a relationship, my career was going great, and everything seemed fine. Now I'm 50 and single. Most personal ads say up to 40 or 45, once in a while to 50. But the culture as a whole seems to say when you're 50, that's it—you're no longer in the market for a relationship. I find this frightening.

So I celebrated turning 50 with an unabashed celebration, as a counter to my tendency to feel unworthy and insecure, that you shouldn't make a big deal out of yourself. I'm really glad I did—it was a landmark event.

Still, being single at 50 feels like my biggest failure, because I'm the kind of guy who should be with someone. Feeling some shame about being single sometimes keeps me from doing things that I might otherwise do—like going to a movie alone or to gay events—I do it anyway, but it doesn't feel that great, because I think I should be there with a partner.

Randy: At this point, partly through AIDS and the gay marriage movement, coupling has become more fashionable. In contrast to the '70s, when gay men in relationships were accused of maintaining their "couples' privilege," the new standard is to be in a relationship with common incomes and a shared vision. Those of us who aren't in a relationship have to fight a sense of being inadequate. Being single, gay, and 50 represents some deficiency.

It's easy to wonder what's wrong with me. What's preventing me from fitting into the mold? Should I compromise more just to settle down? I don't feel like a conscious rebel, not wanting to conform. I'd love to have that special man show up in my life, but I'm not going to try to make someone fit just because it would make life easier. I don't think it would be honest for me unless it was clear that it was going to be mutually beneficial.

On balance, I've missed a good part of a normal human experience by not being in a loving relationship over time, but I've still had a fundamentally happy life. I don't feel like I'm some sad, spinster aunt. I feel quite lucky in having some exceptional friendships. It's not the same as being married, but I've had some of the emotional richness.

There's certainly nothing wrong with being single. And having a relationship is not necessarily an indicator of whether gay men feel happy or content with their lives.[4] Some men feel quite content by themselves—perhaps having sex once in a while with a sex buddy or casual partners, but looking to friends for a sense of connection and emotional intimacy. Anthony Storr, in his book *Solitude: A Return to the Self,* claims that romantic (and even interpersonal) connections have been overrated as sources of meaning and fulfillment.[5] For many people, work, friendship, or spirituality forms the core basis of their sense of meaning in life. In the next example Andrew compares what he's looking for in a relationship with what he can get from friends, traveling, and his spiritual practice.

Andrew: I have a stronger sense of myself, and I feel more content, so I'm not as affected by how people respond to me—not as much as I was when I was younger. In dating situations I swing less from elation to depression. Part of that may be cynicism and protection. But part of that is experience—I have lower expectations about what to expect from a date.

I always had the ideal of finding a life partner. Lately I've been realizing that might never happen. I know there's nothing else I could do to find a relationship that I haven't already tried. I'd prefer to have a relationship, but I can be at peace with it not happening. Because I feel more whole and content within myself, I feel less needy.

I've thought a lot about what a relationship could bring me: companionship and love, and a sense of inner fulfillment. So I asked myself, Where else do I get that? I get it to some extent from friends, when I'm traveling, when I'm in the moment, and when I'm deep in meditation. Instead of just trying to find this one person, why not go to these other sources to get that same experience? Once I realized that these other resources were available, that special person didn't feel so crucial because I could get these things in other ways.

We can always figure out some way to make whatever our current condition is seem totally neurotic: If we're single, it's because we're socially inept or afraid of intimacy. If we long for a relationship, it's because we're insecure. But if we're in a relationship, it's because we're too dependent, and if we want out of a relationship, it's because we're so selfish we can't tolerate the give-and-take that any relationship requires!

It's easy to assume the grass is greener—men in relationships often yearn for the excitement and freedom of "swinging singles," little realizing how isolating it can sometimes feel. And single guys often romanticize what it's like to be in a relationship, not taking into account how all-consuming it can be to deal with another person's foibles and idiosyncrasies. In reality, either road has its joys and sorrows along the way.

Let's be easier on ourselves. If we want a relationship, we can put ourselves out more and get support to sustain our search even though it's difficult at times. If we're ambivalent, we can look at the different interests tugging at us and try to get clear about what we really want. And if we're fairly content being single, we can still make sure that we have quality connections in our lives.

◆   Looking For a Relationship   ◆

Some people say once you stop looking, that's when you find someone—but have you ever tried this with your car keys? You never hear anyone say, "There's really no point in looking for a job—you'll just happen across one someday when you least expect it."

Maybe there's something to be said for being relaxed and interested in one's own pursuits, open to others but without that "lean and hungry" look that scares men away. We don't want to come across as desperate (even if we are)! But it also makes sense to assess for ourselves what it is we're really looking for—not only what we would like in a relationship, but also how we see a relationship fitting into the rest of our lives.

The other extreme is the claim that we can't really love anyone else until we learn to love and accept ourselves. Self-acceptance is a wonderful thing, but it's not as though we have to be totally self-actualized in order to have a relationship! In many ways a relationship can serve to heal and soothe us—but it can also be a source of confrontation with our own deepest conflicts. That doesn't mean that we have to overcome all our neuroses in order to have a relationship; it just means that a relationship commonly presents a more vivid opportunity to confront our demons—which frequently arise in the guise of our partners! However, often as not, the demons we see in our partners are usually our own projections.

In her book *If I'm So Wonderful, Why Am I Still Single?* Susan Page provides some ideas for finding a relationship.[6] I've adapted her steps for finding a mate with some comments that pertain especially to gay men's search for a romantic partner:

Steps for Finding a Relationship
1. What are you looking for in a relationship?
2. Distinguish between desirable and necessary qualities.
3. Make finding a relationship a priority.
4. Come up with a plan that works for you.
5. Put it on your calendar!
6. Remember: Looking for a relationship doesn't have to be fun!
7. Increase your numbers.
8. Be willing to say "No."
9. Don't settle for "better than nothing."
10. Don't stick around with men who are afraid of commitment.
11. Be open to men who don't fit into your usual type.
12. Clarify expectations.

What are you looking for in a relationship?

This is an exercise I've used in my class on gay relationships. By assessing what it is we're really looking for, we can have at least a general idea to guide us in our search. This can include qualities you'd like to find in a partner, but it can also include an assessment of how you'd like to relate to each other. It's helpful to think about what you bring to a relationship as well.

Make a list of these qualities—they can include physical traits, interests, temperament, income, and so on. Don't edit yourself; just put it all down. It may seem too ideal, superficial, or unrealistic, but that's OK. This isn't a final list, or the be-all and end-all of what your future partner has to be like. It's just allowing yourself to get in touch with what you'd really like.

Distinguish between desirable and necessary qualities.

The next step is to go through this list and check off those qualities that are not only desirable, but that you see as essential. Besides physical and sexual attraction, these might include a basic compatibility around lifestyle expectations and a willingness to deal with differences, communicate about feelings, and work through conflicts.

You may find that a lot of aspects you find desirable are not necessarily essential to you. For example, you might like him to be six feet tall and have dark hair and wear glasses and have a mustache. Are all of these qualities absolutely essential? You may prefer that he's hairy, smooth, college-educated, working-class, or interested in art. Or you want him to have a good income and be reliable, sexually spontaneous, and a good listener. Are these essential? They may be—the idea here is not to judge yourself for wanting particular attributes, but to ask yourself what really are the essential qualities that you want in a partner.

Make finding a relationship a priority.

If we want a relationship, it helps to make it a priority. On a scale of one to ten, how much do you want a relationship? "One" could be "content being single," and "ten" could be "totally committed to finding a relationship." This will help you gauge where you stand on this continuum. It's OK to feel ambivalent! Perhaps right now you have other priorities—finishing school, changing jobs, moving to a different city, or even getting over the last relationship. There are many reasons why you may not be ready for a relationship at the present time. Yet even if you're ambivalent, you can still put yourself in situations where you're more likely to encounter other men. You can get some practical experience in a less-pressured environment, and that in itself may influence your readiness for a relationship.

Come up with a plan that works for you.

Forcing yourself to go to bars or dance clubs is not a great plan if you absolutely hate bars and dance clubs. The idea is to come up with a game plan that works for you. What do you enjoy doing anyway that could increase your chances of meeting eligible men?

For example, in most big cities there are many organizations that exist to promote various interests apart from the club scene, such as politics, spirituality, business, sports, arts, and AIDS volunteering. They provide a variety of places to have fun and meet men who share your interests. You can get to know them over time instead of having to decide in one instant whether you want to go to bed with them (and then never see them again!). So you come up with some ideas—visit a group (or start one yourself!), join a dating service, or place an ad. Then…

Put it on your calendar!

This is so important—it's easy for our good intentions to be our last priority: We'll go to this or that event unless something better comes along. Who wouldn't rather go to a movie or out to dinner with a close friend (a sure bet for a fun and stimulating evening) rather than subject himself to the uncertainty of a blind date?

Some men find it helpful to enlist a friend to go with them to an event so they have someone to relate to. When we're active and engaged, we seem a lot more appealing than if we're just standing around waiting for someone to come up and talk to us. The disadvantage of bringing a friend along is that others may assume you're together, so you might want to wander off at times, then come back and talk about how you're doing. You can position yourself so you can see (and make eye contact!) with a prospective interest while looking over your friend's shoulder. You can also provide some encouragement for each other to go up and talk with someone (or even offer to introduce him!).

If you see someone who returns your eye contact, you don't need a witty or clever opening line. All you have to do is smile, say "Hi," and introduce yourself.

Remember: Looking for a relationship doesn't have to be fun!

We have this notion that going out with lots of guys is supposed to be a barrel of monkeys. Then, if we're not having a good time, it's easy to throw our hands in the air and conclude,

"Dating's just not for me." But nobody said this had to be fun.

Comparing dating again with a job search, sure, you'll have times when it isn't pleasant. Going through a job interview can be grueling or boring or humiliating, and so can a blind date. You end up feeling as though you're barking up the wrong tree—but you don't quit trying to find work just because it's not fun anymore.

A belief that Page suggests is that there is someone out there for you and that following through on this plan will lead to finding and establishing a satisfying relationship. Having such a belief can sustain you through the ups and downs and common disappointments that this process involves. Others may be put off by such a leap of faith (or end up blaming themselves if it doesn't work), so try what feels right for you.

Increase your numbers.

If you don't meet many men at work, if you don't like going out, if you end up watching TV on weekends, you're not going to run across very many eligible men. Sure, the FedEx guy may come around once in a while, but dating is a numbers game. The point is to get out there and increase your chances of meeting someone. You can increase your numbers by revising your plan as you go along, experimenting with different groups and situations. Tell your friends you want to meet eligible men, and watch the invitations roll in!

Be willing to say "No."

As mentioned above, you have to be willing to meet a lot of guys to find the one who's right for you. And you never know when someone you meet might have a good friend you'll hit it off with!

Sometimes we inhibit ourselves about going out because we don't know right off whether we really like someone. But just because you go out doesn't mean you have to marry him. Just take it one date at a time. All you have to figure out between now and the next time is whether you want to see him again.

You can increase your numbers by your willingness to say "No" and not get stuck in conversations that keep you from circulating and meeting other eligible men. You don't have to be rude—you can talk for a while, then say "It was nice to talk with you, and I think I'll circulate."

Similarly, you can go out a few times and realize "This isn't for me." Rejection can feel awkward on either end, but it doesn't have to be a big deal. Rather than trying to avoid him with unreturned phone calls, hoping he'll get the message, you can simply let him know that you don't feel any romantic interest, and wish him well. That way you can still be friendly acquaintances rather than feeling awkward or avoiding each other when you run into him again.

Don't settle for "better than nothing."

A corollary to being willing to say "No" is not settling for "better than nothing." Being more self-accepting can help us figure out what we want without constantly undermining ourselves. We don't have to settle for someone who's unreliable, abusive, or demeaning just because we fear being alone. If you're just settling, that will keep you from meeting someone who's really right for you. We can see an involvement with another man as a source of enrichment, not simply as a distraction or a way to feel better about ourselves.

Don't stick around with men who are afraid of commitment.

You think he's great—he's funny, he's handsome, he laughs at your jokes—only he's pretty slow returning calls, he doesn't initiate much contact, and even though he seems glad to hear from you, he's a little vague about the next time he wants to get together. Maybe he's ambivalent, or he just doesn't know how he feels yet.

Now it's true that some people are slow cookers and respond over time to courting. After all, straight men woo women who appear ambivalent at first but gradually warm up to their attention. Gay men, however, tend to disappear at the slightest whiff of rejection.

Some guys are seductive just to boost their own egos and sense of attractiveness but have no intention of following through. Yet they touch that part of ourselves that yearns for closeness, especially in the midst of the self-doubt and vulnerability that we're so likely to feel at midlife. We can be seduced by someone who's gratifying his desire for attention, who then drops us as soon as we express any of our own needs. So don't keep waiting for someone to come around who's not ready for a relationship!

Be open to men who don't fit your usual type.

By distinguishing between desirable and essential qualities, you got an idea as to what type of man you're looking for. Determining which desirable qualities are really essential can help us look beyond our usual "type."

There are lots of different body types that men find attractive—as well as other qualities that we all have to offer besides being a physical type. Having an open heart and feeling a genuine human connection with other men can lead to the willingness to explore intimate connections beyond an initially super-ficial physical attraction.

Many men in long-term relationships say the man they actu-ally ended up with didn't conform to their ideal type of sexual partner. Yet because of his personality and how they hit it off in other ways, they were able to go beyond their usual fantasy to appreciate what this particular man had to offer.

I know that many gay men are skeptical about this. It seems as though it's much easier for women to go beyond the first physical impression and make an emotional connection with a partner that leads to sexual interest, whereas for men it seems to work the other way around. But I don't think this is true for everyone, and it certainly helps, as we get older, to expand be-yond our previous sense of what we found attractive.

If we meet someone who seems nice enough, but we don't feel an initial charge, is it worth sticking around, or are we just settling for "better than nothing"? In other words, what's the difference between a willingness to go beyond your usual type and just "settling"?

The answer to this question lies in assessing the difference between desirable and essential qualities. Sure, your ideal type may be six feet tall with a full head of hair, but what if someone shorter than you whose hair is thinning brought a glimmer to your eye, made you laugh, and stirred something deep inside you? The idea is not to assume that you're better off settling for someone who doesn't really appeal to you—the point is to be aware of the possibility that someone whose picture you might not pick out of a lineup could nonetheless float your boat, ring your bell, or knock your socks off.

Clarify expectations.

When you begin to date, it's helpful to determine at some point whether you're interested in pursuing a relationship—and also whether he's interested in you! Some guys come on so strong, you begin to wonder whether they're really attracted to you or just another warm body. We want to have the sense that someone is relating to us, not just to some image or projection of who they think we are. He may be "in love with love" rather than with you. So be wary of someone who wants to move in on the second date!

Having to know right away whether someone wants to marry you can lead to premature closure—when in doubt, men tend to say "No." Still, it can be maddening to cultivate a relationship with someone over a period of months, looking for nonverbal cues but not even knowing whether he's interested in pursuing a relationship.

There is a lot of ambiguity in gay relationships—you may be interested in finding a partner, but he might just want a sex buddy. We can look for cues, but we can't be expected to read each other's mind. If he seems friendly enough and glad to see you, but you're still not sure where he's coming from, be willing to ask for a reality check: "I've been enjoying getting to know you, but I notice I'm doing most of the initiating, and I wonder what's happening with you."

A few months after our initial interview, Andrew started dating a close friend named Greg. This brought up a lot of issues for him, but the most important one was that he didn't want their exploration of dating to harm their friendship.

Andrew: I had known Greg for a number of years. I had always found him attractive, but he was involved with another man, so the possibility of dating never came up. Even when he broke up with his boyfriend, it didn't really register that he might be available, because by that time we had become friends.

One night we were commiserating about how hard it is to find compatible men to date. Then it occurred to me that we had a lot in common, so why couldn't we date each other? At first it felt more like an intellectual idea—I was open to the possibility but not very attached to it. I figured, what harm could it do, so I decided to check it out.

I said, "Well, we're both attractive, eligible men. We have shared interests in open communication and spirituality. I wouldn't want it to interfere with our friendship, but I've always felt some attraction toward you. So how would you feel about dating?"

He said he didn't want to do anything to interfere with our friendship either, and I figured that was the end of it. But then he said, "I've been attracted to you too. I'd be open to exploring a relationship."

We've taken it real slow—what was important to both of us was that we maintain our friendship and not let dating hurt what we already had. It's over six months now, and I like what's been happening. Since there was some familiarity and stability already there, dating felt like a natural deepening of our friendship. What I really appreciate about this relationship is that we're able to listen and respond to each other's concerns. We enjoy just hanging out, but if something comes up, we can deal with it. My own inner richness, which I've developed through my spiritual practice, is now complemented as well as challenged by my relationship with Greg.

Many men at midlife report a renewed interest in dating. They're less vulnerable where rejection is concerned because they're feeling more content in themselves. And self-confidence has its own attractions. The world of dating can seem intimidating—yet we can also approach it with a sense of adventure and playfulness. As we become more confident about our strengths and what we have to offer, we're in a better position to assess how well we're connecting with another man.

Relating These Themes to Your Own Experience:

- How has your sex life changed?
- What would you like to do differently?
- How do you feel about being single/being in a relationship?
- What are the desirable and essential qualities you'd like in a relationship?
- If you're content being single, what kinds of contact with other men would you like in your life?
- What kind of support can you get to follow through on these ideas?

Notes

1. See *Life Outside* by Michelangelo Signorile. New York: HarperCollins, 1997. Also, *Sexual Ecology: AIDS and the Destiny of Gay Men,* by Gabriel Rotello. New York: Dutton, 1997.
2. A National Sex Panic Summit held in San Diego November

13, 1997, issued a Declaration of Sexual Rights to counter attacks against sexual self-determination. Allan Berube gave a historical perspective on sex panics: "A sex panic is a moral purity crusade. Sex panics usually take place during politically conservative times…and often as a response to the successful political activism of targeted groups…. The media jumps on the bandwagon with lurid exposés, labeling those in the stigmatized group as dangerous perverts, deviants, or degenerates who need to be identified, controlled, and contained with drastic action to restore order and protect society." See "Sex Panics in History" by Allan Berube, *The Harvard Gay and Lesbian Review,* spring 1998.

3. *The Farewell Symphony* by Edmund White recounts a fast-paced whirl of momentary encounters in New York during the '70s. New York: Knopf, 1997. At the Sex Panic conference, Allan Berube described "creative moments of intimate sexual adventure with strangers I never saw again. These erotic spaces have been little utopias of Whitmanesque camaraderie—places where I could imagine living in a world that deeply valued the varieties of erotic desire among men." (See note 2.)

4. "HIV serostatus, or relationship status as single or coupled, may not be strongly linked to any particular resolution of being gay and becoming older." Robert Kertzner, "Entering Midlife: Gay Men, HIV, and the Future." *Journal of the Gay and Lesbian Medical Association,* June 1997.

5. *Solitude: A Return to the Self* by Anthony Storr. New York: Free Press, 1988.

6. *If I'm So Wonderful, Why Am I Still Single?* by Susan Page. New York: Viking, 1988.

CHAPTER 7

IMPACT OF MIDLIFE ON GAY RELATIONSHIPS

Some gay men have long-term relationships starting in their 20s or 30s, and bonds begun at this stage of life can be very gratifying. At midlife they may begin to question where their relationship is headed—whether they still have the same goals, mutual attraction, and shared interests. In this chapter we'll look at some of the effects of midlife on gay relationships.

◆ How Relationships Change Over Time ◆

In their book *The Male Couple: How Relationships Develop*, David McWhirter and Andrew Mattison outline a number of stages that the couples in their study seemed to pass through over time.[1] With any description of stages, it's important to realize that this is a generalization of what was seen in a particular group at a certain point in time—it is not intended as a pre-scription of how your relationship should develop. Yet it can be a relief to see how some of the issues that are emerging in your relationship may be reflected in the experiences of other couples.

Stage One—Blending (year one)
- Merging
- Limerence (romantic love)
- Equalizing of partnership
- High sexual activity

Stage Two—Nesting (years two and three)
- Homemaking
- Finding compatibility
- Decline of limerence (romantic love)
- Ambivalence

Stage Three—Maintaining (years four and five)
- Reappearance of the individual
- Risk-taking
- Dealing with conflict
- Establishing traditions

Stage Four—Building (years six through ten)
- Collaborating
- Increasing productivity
- Establishing independence
- Dependability of partners

Stage Five—Releasing (years 11 through 20)
- Trusting
- Merging of money and possessions
- Constricting
- Taking each other for granted

Stage Six—Renewing (beyond 20 years)
- Achieving security
- Shifting perspectives
- Restoring the partnership
- Remembering

Each developmental stage can be understood as a potential crisis in the relationship: whether to move in together; how to deal with parents and other relatives; whether to allow outside sexual partners; or how to deal with finances. If members of a couple find that what they want is too different, they may decide to go their separate ways. However, a resolution of differences that takes the needs and desires of both partners into consideration can result in a deepened commitment to their relationship.

Age Differences

In Mattison's and McWhirter's study, some of the men who had been together the longest had the largest age differences between them.[2] They surmised that age difference is one source of tension that helps the couple maintain interest in one another.

The stages outlined above may express themselves differently in a relationship where there is a significant age difference. The older man may be seen as a mentor in the beginning of a relationship, offering guidance and assistance. The younger man may appreciate his help, but as he grows older, he establishes himself in his own career and develops other interests. This causes a shift in their previous roles, and he may resent being treated as an inexperienced youth. The older man may be surprised by this resentment, especially after all the sacrifices he has made to help the younger man get established. If they can understand the significant alteration in roles that has taken place between them, they can still value the memory of how they used to be together, even as they adjust to seeing one another as peers.

Antoine is 19 years younger than his lover, Bill. They've been together for 23 years. Antoine describes the transition that has taken place in their relationship over the years.

Antoine: I was 22 when I first met Bill. Now I'm 45. I was dependent on him way back then emotionally, for sex, for everything. He was the leader—he'd take the initiative about what was happening in our lives, and I just tagged along.

Over the years our roles have changed. Now I have an accounting degree, and I feel more like an equal at a professional level. In terms of who's guiding our relationship, I'm an equal there, too. It's easier for me to say I don't want to do this, let's do something else. Back in '76, I would never do that. Emotionally, though, I'm still dependent on him. I don't know what I'd do if he wasn't around.

Another source of tension in couples with significant age differences is the discrepancy between their sexual desires. A decline in frequency of sexual relations is common with most couples after the first couple of years. This is true with couples of similar age as well. However, the older man may already have experienced a decline in his desire for sex, and this can cause some frustration and tension between him and his partner. Openly acknowledging this difference is an important first step in trying to figure out how they want to deal with differing desires.

Victor: My lover is 16 years younger and has more sexual energy than I do, but we've found ways to manage that in our relationship. We've been together six years, and the initial fire of sexuality inevitably burns down. Yet both of us still have a high need for physical contact and cuddling.

I don't know if the change in my sexuality is part of midlife or simply the result of this particular relationship. I've always wanted to create a certain quality of connection. Sex became a path for creating intimacy, and now I have a connection that is amazingly satisfying. So sex is relatively minor, but we're still very physically affectionate. It's unusual for us not to spend the whole night totally wrapped up together.

Individuation

One of the most significant sources of conflict that I have seen in gay relationships comes after the initial blending and nesting stages, when one partner begins to develop interests outside of the relationship. The other partner may feel threatened by this apparent distancing. Up until this shift, they may have spent a lot of time together, nurturing their sense of being a couple.

This reemergence of the individual is a natural development in any relationship, but not everyone has the same timing. One partner may be ready to reclaim his sense of being an individual, while the other needs reassurance that they are still creating a life together. The one who seeks other interests may feel guilty and resentful, while the other wonders what's wrong or feels rejected.

This natural conflict can be further complicated if they are not able to talk about their differences. The man who feels rejected may become jealous of his partner's other interests, while the one who wants more space in the relationship becomes secretive about his activities. This conflict can intensify as each partner's effort to meet his own needs elicits a corresponding escalation in his partner: the more one pulls away, the more his partner needs expressions of affection, leading the other to distance himself even further.

Recognizing that the reemergence of the individual is an expectable and even healthy development in a relationship can help both partners realize that just because one or both of them wants to develop other interests, this does not necessarily mean they no longer value the relationship. They may need to find ways to reassure each other even as they begin to explore separate interests or friendships.

Kevin: I need my own company much more than I did when I was young. I used to find it hard to be alone. My dream was that I'd meet someone and six months later we'd live together. Now I accept that with my personality, I don't want to live with my partner. I love mingling our worlds when we're together, but I need solitude in a way I never did before.

Antoine: Because my partner is so unpredictable, there's always uncertainty. I've learned to live with that. What we'll do on any given day—whether we're going to a movie or going out to eat—getting him to focus is hard. He starts projects, then changes. He wanted to be a world-famous photographer—now he's building aquariums. I have a closet full of camera equipment. Things change. It wasn't all right for a while, but it's easier for me now.

Countering Boredom

Another common complaint is boredom. Couples end up feeling that they know each other almost too well. Daily interactions have become perfunctory, and they begin to avoid each other.

Boredom may signal their need to individuate. By recognizing the underlying feelings of frustration, they can talk about their need to explore other interests. Sharing different interests often revives the relationship by giving them something to talk about once they get back together. Increasing their toleration of differences can actually enhance their capacity for intimacy.

While it's helpful to look at ways to enliven a relationship that has gone stale, boredom is not always the result of too much familiarity. In many of the couples I've worked with, boredom can also result from the denial of conflict and from the effort it takes to suppress the tension between them. Couples who have been frightened by the open expression of conflict may avoid controversial topics and suppress their true feelings. Over time, larger and larger areas of their lives become off-limits because it doesn't really feel safe to acknowledge or talk about them. When you can't talk about what's really going on between you, it's easy for daily contact to feel perfunctory, stale, and boring.

Some couples decide to embark on some major project together as a way to revitalize their relationship. They may buy a house that needs renovation or start a business together. This may resemble a heterosexual couple's attempt to rekindle their relationship by having a child. Having a common goal or project can be a wonderful way to engage with each other, but if they haven't dealt with underlying conflicts, their conflict may express itself through difficulties in their project. Or, if they are able to use the new venture to suppress their conflicts, they become depressed once the project is finished. The house is finally refurbished, the new business is going, or the partner finishes graduate school, then the couple splits up.

Many people attribute such breakups to the stresses that accompany such all-consuming projects, and these stresses should not be minimized. However, the project may also serve the function of suppressing underlying differences that the couple has difficulty facing directly. A similar dynamic can be seen in heterosexual couples who split up after the children have left home.

The idea, then, is to be willing to bring up differences and address conflicts, but in a way that strengthens the relationship rather than damaging it. Instead of blaming each other, you can recognize that you have a difference and listen to each other's underlying desires. Then try to find a solution that takes both partners' needs into consideration.[3]

Open Relationships

Some couples who have previously been monogamous decide at some point to open their relationship to sexual affairs. They may realize they have different sexual interests, and rather than looking to each other, they try having sex outside the relationship. For some couples, this seems to enliven their own time together. For others, it can become a threat, and they need to renegotiate their agreements to safeguard their own relationship. Some couples find that they gradually drift apart sexually and become more like roommates. Others may experiment for a while, then find that outside relationships detract from their own level of intimacy and decide to close the relationship again. And some couples find a way to keep communicating about what's coming up for them even as they continue to have outside sexual contacts. Specific agreements may shift and change, but their commitment to each other is maintained over time.

A more recent development with HIV-negative men involves having unprotected sex within a monogamous relationship, following two negative antibody results six months apart. The important component of this agreement is that if there is any unprotected sex outside the relationship, they agree to inform each other and begin using protection until they can retest again twice. It should also be agreed that telling your partner you had unprotected sex should not be grounds for ending the relationship, since that would inhibit disclosure. This kind of agreement obviously takes a high level of trust, maturity, and willingness to be forthcoming about emotionally difficult matters.

Not every relationship fits into a standard mold. Gay men have been very creative in forming many kinds of relationships, and the nature of these relationships may shift over time. Victor has known Gary for 26 years, and they bought a house together 15 years ago. They started out as lovers but later became friends who still share a very close bond—yet there is room for each of them to have other relationships. Victor has been with his current lover for six years, and explains how this has worked out with Gary.

Victor: There are more forms of relationships than we have names to describe them. We have language for lover, for friend, for husband, for certain relationships, but there are a lot more possibilities. The real transformation with Gary, by far my most significant long-term relationship, has been a recognition that our relationship is what it is. It doesn't lend itself to a particular name. Simply to acknowledge and appreciate what it is, is incredible.

This grasping notion that there can only be one primary relationship, when there is a real complexity in life, can make it tough. With Curtis, my former lover, we had this tremendous crisis over whether our relationship was primary or my relationship with Gary was primary. It's just a word. That's what got us hung up—to believe that this word has a transcendent meaning.

Gary and I have gotten smarter over the years. We're closer now than we've ever been over the 26 years that we've been together. And the reason is that we've finally evolved to place where we've accepted our relationship for exactly what it is.

I'm devoted to him. I'd do anything for him—even lay down my life for him. We're completely intertwined, and it would never occur to me to make a life-changing decision without consulting him. He's my best friend who I can count on so thoroughly I don't even have to think about it. Will we survive what's going to happen next? I don't think about that with Gary any more than I would think about my right hand. Of course, if it got cut off, that would be a loss, but I think of him as that close.

My current lover was 22 when we met. The first month was uncomfortable—I wondered whether he would be able to accept my relationship with Gary. But he got what our relationship was right away. Rather than seeing it as a threat, he realized that I was a person who was capable of a long-term, committed relationship.

◆   Renewal or Leaving?   ◆

I have seen a number of clients over the years who were struggling with whether to stay in a relationship that had a lot of unresolved problems. On one hand, it seemed tempting to leave. On the other, they had already invested a lot of time and effort, and were reluctant to just let it go. Whether a relationship is capable of renewal or it's better to leave is a very personal decision. So it's helpful to consider some of the following issues in making a decision about whether to leave or stay.

Signs To Look For:

Is your restlessness due to your own unresolved midlife issues?

Have you spoken up about the behavior that bothers you or talked about what's missing?

Is your partner willing to engage with you about the problems you see in the relationship, or does he dismiss your concerns, claiming it's "your problem"?

Is he willing to join you in couples counseling?

Has your partner refused treatment for alcohol or substance abuse?

Do your conflicts escalate into put-downs, sarcasm, or other emotional abuse?

Has your partner used threats of suicide or violence to control you?

Have you ever been shoved, slapped, hit, or threatened with physical violence? (I do not recommend couples counseling for domestic violence, as it tends to escalate the violence unless the batterer has accepted responsibility for the violence, sought treatment, and learned how to handle his anger more constructively.)

HIV can have a profound influence on the decision whether to leave or stay. Men whose partners are HIV-positive may base this decision on a sense of responsibility to their partner, or they may be motivated by guilt. HIV-positive men may find that what they're willing to put up with shifts as their health improves and they feel more optimistic about their prospects for the future.

Kevin: One big dilemma I had was whether to stay in a relationship with a man I knew would die before me or to use the real difficulties in the relationship as a reason to leave. I had an older friend who recognized how much I loved Sam. He had been through the experience of entering a relationship with someone who was HIV-positive. He was able to tell me that even though he knew his lover would die, it was the best five years of his life. I would have left that relationship if it hadn't been for this friendship and his words of advice.

Tony: Before I went back to school, I was with my lover for 12 years, and I question whether we would have stayed together if he had been healthy. We had grown apart in different ways. He'd become this staid businessman, into his career, with a more traditional approach to life, and I wasn't like that.

I took my career seriously, but he'd come home and watch TV, and thought of himself as a middle-aged fart. I liked to go out, go for a hike, take vacations more adventuresome than a gay cruise. Trekking in Nepal would be more to my liking. So I questioned this at the time: Do I want to be with a guy who goes to work, comes home, and turns on the TV, and who no longer takes care of his body or cares about dressing well? He'd be content wearing the same plastic raincoat his father wore. But when he got sick, I wasn't going to leave him. I still loved him and took care of him until the end.

The next example concerns Brian and Jason, who had been together for six years. Jason was very domestic—he liked to cook and refinish furniture, and he helped remodel Brian's house. But for Brian, something was missing—he assumed it was because Jason wasn't the right partner for him. After they broke up he wondered whether he had displaced his midlife dilemma onto Jason—rather than confronting what was missing from his own life, he decided to leave the relationship.

Brian: After six years Jason wanted a commitment. But I asked, "What are we committing to?" He said, "Two people are just stuck together."

I found this devastating. I didn't want to hear that, and yet now it sounds wise, in a way. Wendell Berry compared marriage to poetry. A marriage is like working within the structure of a poetic form. You stick to the form because it's something you've decided to work within. It limits you in some ways, but it also allows you to explore other aspects that may never have occurred to you if you didn't have to stay within those limits. Marriage is like that too.

So when Jason said you're just stuck together, this was his own blunt, but wise way of saying what Berry said. See what you can make of it, for better or worse.

I should have asked myself, What was my relationship keeping me from doing? I could have done a better job of figuring this out with Jason. I feel more humble now about what it takes to be in a relationship. There are things I could have learned from him and grown from.

I left Jason after asking him, "What's the point in our staying together?" I should have been asking this about myself: What was the point now, to my own life? I displaced my midlife dilemma onto the relationship, and left it without really working this through. I see it as a *puer* decision to chuck it rather than going into therapy and trying to figure out what it was I was really looking for. I may have come up with the same answer about leaving the relationship, but because I saw the relationship as the problem rather than my own quandary, something was left unfinished. By leaving Jason without working through this, I kept wondering whether I made the right choice, and I still had to come to terms with my own sense of drift and lack of meaning.

I still experience an irreconcilable ambivalence. Emotionally and domestically we were very close, and I could imagine going back to try again. But on the other hand, there was a level of intellectual and political stimulation that I never had with him, and I couldn't imagine the next 20 years having dinner together and just not having that much to talk about. It's still a source of painful conflict and ambivalence.

My parents didn't talk about anything that profound at dinner, yet they seemed deeply satisfied with each other. Jason was very interested in the home sphere, how we could redecorate, or who said what to whom at work. But I like to talk about the big questions—politics, the cosmos, and the meaning of life.

He's since gotten involved with someone else, and now he lives right around the corner, so maybe as neighbors we're just right.

It's not an easy decision either to end a long-term relationship or to stay and struggle. It's easy to see the relationship as the source of the problem, yet relationship conflict can also be stimulated by unresolved midlife issues.

There is often a lot at stake in a decision to leave or stay in a long-term relationship, both financially and emotionally. The idea is to sort through what's coming up for you, as well as what's going on between you and your partner. Then see if he's willing to engage with you to explore your feelings, sort through your options, and determine whether you want to renew your commitment. It's also helpful to remember that just because a relationship doesn't last forever doesn't necessarily mean it was a "failure."

◆   Creating Our Own Families   ◆

Many gay men have created their own extended families of choice through their relationships and friendships. Significant friendships form some of the most important relationships that many of us have. AIDS has taken a devastating toll on our social networks, and it takes effort to reestablish friendships that last over time.

At midlife a feeling of loss regarding not having children may stimulate the desire in some gay men to become involved with child-rearing.[4] Some men have children from a previous heterosexual marriage, while others decide to have their own children as openly gay men—either with lesbian friends or through adoption. Other men make connections with children through friends, big brother and mentor programs, or foster parenting.

Randy: I'm crazy about children. Although I'm glad I didn't get married just to have children, I regret that I haven't had the sustained relationship with children that parents have. I've tried through friends and with my nieces and nephews. Having a connection with young people is an important part of our humanity.

Brian: In the first half of my life, career and relationship were my main focus. I tried a few jobs before settling on my current career, and had two or three significant relationships. Then I found myself at midlife and single, with my career going well and still wanting a relationship, but neither of those seemed like enough. So I began looking around for something else to do—having a child, writing a book, or starting a second career.

My biggest decision at midlife was to become a father. I see raising my son as a gigantic project for the whole rest of my life. What's the purpose of life? What's the second half of my life going to look like? Whatever the questions were, he's now a major part of the answer. I hope this was not the only reason—to get out of my midlife crisis—but in the course of my analysis, I sorted through how much I wanted to be a father.

Tony: It wasn't just a rational decision to have a child, weighing pros and cons. I always had a sense that I would have children, it was an expectation that I grew up with. When I was 27 I met a guy who fathered a child as a gay man, and I knew that would be me. It was just a matter of finding the person to do it with.

I thought about the repercussions on the child. I wanted to protect him from the social stigma and envisioned sending him to a private school in Berkeley with alternative families. But I didn't anticipate the downside—what an incredible struggle it would be, and how much pain it would cause in my own life. Soon after our son was born, the women I had him with reneged on our agreement. The custody battle that ensued was extremely painful and lasted a number of years until we finally worked things out to coparent in a cooperative way.

I felt that the most important thing we have is love. A feeling of self-worth can develop in a child if he's nurtured in the right way. I figured I could help him develop the tools he needs to become a loving person and contribute to society. But my son had a lot of problems as a young child. We felt a lot of pain and guilt, wondering if we somehow did this to him. We finally discovered that he's hyperactive and has a learning disability. Now that we're successfully dealing with these problems, he's a lot happier.

Having a child immersed me in a heterosexual world, which was not comfortable for me at the time. I was surrounded by macho dads and traditional families. I had to learn how to relate to them with integrity as an openly gay man. That was hard, and I've grown a lot.

I used to feel that a father needs to be good at sports, things I'm not good at. But now I'm fine with telling my son I'm not into sports, and if you want that we can find activities for you to participate in. I have other things to offer, like reading stories and traveling, and I feel comfortable giving him those, even if they're traditionally more "feminine."

He's in the third grade, and the child of the week gets to talk about his family. When it was his turn, he brought in pictures and told the class his mother is a lesbian and his father is gay. The school bully later called him the "son of lesbians." We talked with him about how people have prejudices. The school was supportive, he seemed OK with it, and there have been no other incidents.

Many gay couples have grown old together in the past, but we have not had very many examples in the media of older gay couples who feel good about themselves and have a lively network of other gay friends. Yet it appears that gay couples who survive the common changes that occur as they progress through various stages are able to deepen their affection and caring for one another. To know that you are able to love and be loved and to trust that you will be there for each other can be very gratifying. You develop a sense of trust and assurance that whatever difficulties you may encounter in the future, you'll face them together.

A key to long-term couples' success seems to be their ability to communicate about their differences.[5] The resilience that develops through experience is reinforced by their expression of genuine affection. Their feelings are kept alive by their willingness to support each other in their own personal growth.

Relating These Themes to Your Own Experience

- What do you want now from a relationship? How has that changed since you first came out?
- If you're in a relationship now (or looking at a past relationship), how has it changed over time?
- What else would you like?
- What happens when you express your desires?

Notes

1. *The Male Couple: How Relationships Develop* by David McWhirter and Andrew Mattison (Englewood Cliffs, N.J.: Prentice-Hall, 1984), pp. 16-17.
2. All of the couples in their study who were together for longer than 30 years (eight couples) had an age difference of between

five and 16 years. *The Male Couple,* p. 286.

3. For suggestions on resolving conflicts and improving commu-
    nication skills in gay relationships, see *Love Between Men* by
    Rik Isensee. Los Angeles: Alyson, 1996.

4. "The Psychological Adaptations of Middle-Aged Gay Men
    to Being Childless," by K. Farrell. Master's Thesis, California
    State University, Long Beach, Calif., December 1992. (Cited
    by Robert Kertzner in *Textbook of Homosexuality.* See note 11,
    Chapter 10.)

5. "Can We Talk? Can We Really Talk? Communication as a
    Key Factor in the Maturing Homosexual Couple," by John
    Alan Lee. *Gay Midlife and Maturity,* edited by John Alan Lee,
    pp. 143-155. New York: Haworth Press, 1991.

CHAPTER 8

LOSS AND MORTALITY

Becoming aware of our mortality is a common midlife theme, and this awareness has been accelerated for most gay men by the specter of AIDS.[1] Midlife is also a time when many people get in touch with previous losses, which include not only people, but lost opportunities and dreams. In this chapter we'll look at the effects of such losses and what it means to come to terms with our own mortality.

Brian: I never used to understand why novelists write so much about death. Now I'm more aware of the brevity of life, and it makes total sense. Death is a container that puts everything else in perspective—the fact that one's life ends means that everything you do is important—or not important at all. Experiencing that paradox—that's what it means to "live with one's death as an adviser," as Carlos Casteneda describes it.

In my 20s I felt like there was always plenty of time to do everything. Then there came a moment when I realized I have a finite number of good years left to do whatever I want to do.

The crux of midlife is the realization that time is running out.

Andrew: I'm always aware of my mortality, through the AIDS crisis. Part of it is a fear of the unknown and loss of control. Stephen Levine says how we die is determined by how we live our lives. You either struggle and have a bad time, or you learn to go with it. Fighting it isn't pretty. I'm trying to go with it more in my life.

Tony: I've always assumed I would die young. My father died at 56 of a massive heart attack; his father and uncle died at the same age. I always felt the same thing would happen to me. In college I figured so what, that seemed so far away—I still had my whole life ahead of me. Now 56 doesn't seem that distant.

I still have the sense that I won't live that long. Getting old is not in keeping with the way I've lived my life. I'm not very cautious; I often do what feels good, fuck the future. I figured when I turned 40 I'd start worrying about coronary disease, clean up my diet, but I haven't done that. I eat a lot of pizza and ice cream. I exercise my body, but probably not in a way that's good for my joints. I get the payoff of an OK-looking body, but I'm not paying attention to what that may do down the line.

I don't really fear death so much. I expect it to be sudden, not something I have to deal with. I won't know what hit me. That's a comfort. The idea of being sick for years or having a stroke and being dependent would be hideous to me.

Hal: From my spiritual sense, death is just a transition. Maybe the other side is another incarnation—unless you decide this is the last one—which is what I'm hoping for. It's not the death that concerns me; it's injuring the body, the experience of pain between living and dying, even though I know that on the other side it's OK.

Mario: I love the idea of dying. I saw David and Carl and a lot of other friends die. I feel that I'm looking forward to death, not as something horrible. I hope I'm conscious enough to be present with it.

Steve: I don't think of myself as afraid of death, but then I felt a gut-level anxiety over a recent brush with possible HIV. Death no longer seemed abstract. But I think my anxiety is related not so much to death as debilitation. There's a freeing aspect to death—it helps me remind myself, what does it matter what people think if I'm going to die.

◆   HIV and Multiple Loss   ◆

The current generation of gay men at midlife has been decimated by AIDS, and the loss of so many long-term friends and lovers has been devastating. There is no way to replace lifelong relationships—all the friends who shared our early experiences of coming out, having sex, going to demonstrations, traveling across the country, partying with roommates, and staying up half the night talking about the meaning of life. So many of the friends and lovers who shared our youthful triumphs and disappointments and were always there—are there no longer.

Multiple loss has caused some men to "numb out," retreat from contact, and become further depressed because of their isolation. We can come to terms with significant losses by allowing ourselves to grieve and by reaching out for support.

Antoine: My best friends from high school and college and the first man I had sex with all died from AIDS. They were all my age. Sometimes it's difficult because I feel like they left me behind. I miss them. I'll be driving somewhere, and something will remind me of them. I cry a lot easier, and sometimes I'll pull over to the side of the road.

Mario had always been a fun-loving guy, getting high and partying with his friends. But then his lover's worsening condition compelled him to make a conscious choice about being emotionally present in his role as his lover's caretaker.

Mario: I am not a young man anymore. I'm not 20. I'm a man, and I love that maturity and responsibility. It was kind of thrust upon me with David's health. I needed to be responsible, and I wanted to fulfill that role well. I think that's what being an adult is—doing the best you can and understanding what you can't do.

When David got sick I chose to be his caregiver. I was smoking a lot of pot, getting high, and one night I called him from a party and he asked me to come home, he was just diagnosed with CMV. He'd go blind unless he started this new treatment, and needed to talk.

I was totally high. I realized that even though I was there physically, I couldn't focus my mind to be emotionally present. That was the day I stopped smoking pot. I realized I can't go through this by removing myself, I have to be in it. Making that decision made everything special between us. We had some good moments which would never have happened if I'd been zoned out on pot. I see that as a choice of growing up.

◆ Grieving ◆

Whatever grief and pain we avoided in youth we often have to face again at midlife: disappointments we experienced while growing up and the lack of a supportive culture when we were first coming out. These memories can be restimulated later by rejections from other gay men.

Sources of grief can include missed opportunities, losses, and disappointments in our careers or other lifelong goals. Grief also involves confronting our fading looks, the loss of sexual stamina, and the loss of attention we may have received because of our youthful charms.

The reason this may come up again at this time is that we can more clearly recognize the profound nature of our losses. As boys we may have been so preoccupied with survival that we couldn't really let it sink in. It would have been too distracting from our tasks as young men. Yet once we're through struggling, we can see more clearly what else might have been, and we begin to grieve for that loss.

Hal: When I didn't go to medical school or become a writer or go into the artificial intelligence field—sometimes I think there's a whole life that died, and I grieve for that part of me that is no longer there. Giving up those dreams of what I could have been. That's why the current moment is so intense—I'm not willing to give this one up.

Steve: I've done a lot of grieving, for the breakup of my relationship, for the problem with my hands, not being able to swim or work out or even do gardening. I sometimes grieve for lost opportunities. I didn't party much in youth. I actually had more lost opportunities in adolescence than I do now.

Andrew: Death started in my life when I was 20. I've had significant losses all through my life. I was pretty closed down for a long time, not letting it in, not wanting to feel it. Now I feel more open to my emotions and more affected by loss and death. Even though I know that's what life is—people are born, people die—I miss some people who were very close to me. I'm not sure if I have more acceptance about it now, or if I'm still in denial and shut down.

Victor: I had more losses five years ago than I do now, but I'm getting better at it. Buddhism teaches that it's the unwillingness to let go that creates pain. When it's possible to accept the loss, that's what can finally release the pain.

When I'm not in my right mind, old dreams that seem like they're gone can emerge again, like being rich and famous or even having some coherence and stability and permanence. I know that's all nonsense. I can complain that this is not the way things were supposed to turn out, things were supposed to be better than this, but that just keeps me stuck.

Mario: Certain times of the year, I'm moody, and then realize it's the anniversary of someone's death. As time goes on it becomes less intense. But it's always there, and when it comes up I allow myself to grieve. I don't see AIDS movies that often, but when I do see one, I don't stop the tears. I saw *Hercules* and even got choked up in that. It's great to be watching a cartoon and get teary-eyed.

The memories are always there. Probably it's worse because we've seen so many people die so young. David would be 42—he didn't even make it to 40. After years of being so focused on David's health, it's nice not to have to make those critical decisions—do I stay or do I go? Would I get involved in another relationship with someone who has HIV? Of course, I'm involved with friends who have AIDS, but they're not my lovers. I'd have to cross that bridge when I got to it.

◆   New Hopefulness   ◆

With the advent of protease inhibitors and other drugs coming down the pike, there's a new hopefulness that AIDS may at last become a manageable, chronic illness, if not be cured altogether. At the time of this writing, it is still unknown whether reducing the virus to undetectable levels will result in its eventual eradication. And there are some men who haven't responded to these new treatments. There is also some concern that drug-resistant strains may survive and begin to attack the immune system again. But in the meantime, death rates have fallen, and great numbers of men who had previously retired from work or gone on disability now face the prospect of moving on with their lives.

Before the development of these treatments, for many HIV-positive men, midlife had seemed somewhat irrelevant. They lived the last few years as though there would be no future. It was important to do things now, rather than waiting. Many have given up their jobs and cashed in their life insurance.

Now, with T-cells over 200, no opportunistic infections, and undetectable virus levels, some men may no longer qualify for disability. Despite the great news, this new hopefulness has precipitated a crisis for many men who have to deal with this in-between status—feeling much better physically, but with few guarantees that if they go off disability, they'd be able to get back on in case of recurring illness.

Kevin: One HIV-positive friend was a workaholic, has been on disability, and now in his late 40s is beginning to realize he may live for a while. Many other HIV-positive men who have been out of work don't want to go back to their old lives. For people who think they might die soon, life becomes so precious, it's hard to imagine spending time in a meaningless job.

The reality that I'm going to die one day comes to me more often than it used to. When I reached 35 I thought at least I won't die young, and that was a relief. Now it's weird to think I may die of something besides AIDS. It seems a lonelier thing to die of something else. So many others were dying of AIDS, you were a part of something. Now the idea that I could die of some other disease or accident seems odd. It's like my AIDS death anxiety has been replaced by a more normal vision of decline. I'll die like everyone else rather than as a person with AIDS.

Because of HIV, I've lived with uncertainty since '81. I still don't like it, but I've managed to have a fulfilling life even with the uncertainty that being HIV-positive brings. Maybe being positive all these years has made midlife seem pretty trivial. At 40 most men are just beginning to be aware they're going to decline, but I started living that way at 25.

Because I'm HIV-positive, I've lived with death every day for the last 15 years. I'm not bitter; I've been doing this for a long time—adjusting to the potential for death and decline in the near term. At 35 I was happy to be alive, and now I'm 41. I expected to be dead by now. Instead of being a period of reconciliation to limits, or adjusting, it's like spring again. So at the same time I'm going through the decline of middle age, I have the feeling that I'm going to live. Instead of waiting to die, I have a new sense that I have a future. It's very powerful. Maybe that's why I'm happy in midlife. I'm never bored, and I have a full life. I'm sure that has to do with being HIV-positive. No question.[2]

◆   Dealing With Aging Parents   ◆

Watching our parents decline through their later years brings home the reality of our own aging process. It often brings about a shift in our caretaking responsibilities. Aging parents can become somewhat childlike in their dependency and need for care, so a role reversal often takes place at this time of life.

Many of us felt rejected by our fathers because of our homosexuality. Then we rejected the rejection, which often led to estrangement. At midlife we may get in touch with the basis of our loss—the longing many of us felt to be closer to our fathers. Mourning for that loss allows us to come to terms with what was missing, and we no longer feel as vulnerable. We discover that we can reach out to other men for nurturing and healing. By healing ourselves, something starts to shift in our relationship with our fathers—we may no longer feel the need to oppose our fathers or prove ourselves. We may still not be able to talk about significant issues, but some of us find a way to be around each other that feels different than when we were younger.

For men whose parents never really came to terms with their homosexuality, the reversal in roles can create a transformation in attitudes and a letting go of previous expectations on both sides. Some parents begin to appreciate what their son has to offer, and the son's sense of self-worth is firmly enough in place that he no longer has such a strong need for explicit signs of approval, recognition, or even acceptance. He may have taken a stand at various times when he was younger, but at midlife there's often less of a need to prove himself, because he's already established his own identity. Some men have partners of many years who are considered part of the family, even if there has never been an open acknowledgment of their relationship. They may develop a sense of mutual respect and caring, despite their parents' reluctance to openly embrace a "gay lifestyle." As Mario indicates in the following example, some of these attitudes also vary according to a family's cultural values.

Mario: I'm out to my family, but like most Latin families, that's something we don't talk about. Out of respect for them, I don't cause scenes or make demands in their home. In the same way, I don't hide anything when they come to visit me. For example, I didn't bring my lover home, but he met my mother when she came to visit me.

I came out to my mother and thanked her for her support while David was dying. She said, "I've always known—I just didn't think you wanted to talk about it." I still don't want to talk about "being gay" with her, although I'll refer to whomever I'm seeing.

Brian: I watch my mother responding to my baby. She cannot tolerate the fact that life is moving on. The structure of families is undergoing radical change, and I'm part of that. She doesn't know how to relate to her grandson if it's not in the context of a heterosexual marriage. Roles are changing, and she doesn't know what her role is. Her response to changing roles is to conserve social institutions in a form she finds familiar. She can't tolerate the constant flux of life.

Many people assume that you get more conservative as you grow older. I see conservatism as a denial of death—you want things to stay the way they are. Which is comforting, because the fantasy is that when I die things won't change. So death loses its sting, since things will continue on the same way they always have. The reality is that life will go on changing in the future at an even greater rate, in ways we can't even imagine. To accept one's death really means that we will miss out on a whole lot. You meet people in their 70s who seem "young at heart." I think what we mean by that is that they are open to the fact that life is still changing, and it will go on doing so even after they're gone.

Victor: A current loss—my mother will probably live to 100, she's in such good shape she walks faster than me. She's now in her mid 70s, and she's losing her memory. The last couple of months, the idea of losing a very important person, even though she would still be there, has been difficult.

I grew up with traditional Portuguese parents, and the mother is the central figure in the family. The loss of the mother in my culture is very profound. We were emotionally very open— I saw my father cry; I never had it in my head that men didn't cry—and family members were very affectionate with each other. My mother stands for all that. So it's a real loss not to have her in that central role anymore.

Kevin: Losing parents is a big change at midlife. The death and decline of parents is much easier for people who have found a way to be on good terms with them. When my father died, that was untraumatic, but I can already sense that it will be a big adjustment in my world when my mother dies. I know I'll do an entire review of our relationship in therapy. I'll probably regret not spending more time with her.

With the death of my mother, a psychological safety net will no longer be there. The idea that no matter what happens, you can go home, will disappear. I'm sure I'll adjust to the awareness, but I will be significantly more alone in the world than I am now. I would be glad for my mother to die before me, because I'm HIV-positive, and I think it would be terrible for her to bury me. I think it's terrible for any mother to bury a child.

After all that we've been through with AIDS, facing our own mortality may not seem like such a big crisis. But what it does for many men is to focus their attention on what's really important. In the next chapter we'll look at the role of work in our quest for meaning at midlife.

Relating These Themes to Your Own Experience:

- What sort of losses have you experienced?
- How has AIDS affected you?
- Are there friends, groups, or other sources that you'd like to reach out to for increased support?
- What is your relationship now with your parents?
- What else would you want?
- If they have already passed away, what do you wish they could have known about you?

Notes

1. In "Midlife, Gay Men, and the AIDS Epidemic," Robert Hopcke describes how the confrontation with mortality caused by AIDS can contribute to an "AIDS-induced midlife." *Quadrant* 35 (1): pp. 101-109, 1992.

2. In "Entering Midlife: Gay Men, HIV, and the Future," Robert Kertzner also cites this renewed sense of possibilities

at midlife, a time when most men are confronted with diminished expectations. *Journal of the Gay and Lesbian Medical Association*, June 1997.

CHAPTER 9

MEANINGFUL WORK

Love and work—Freud identified these two areas as the main sources of life's meaning and satisfaction. Especially for men, work has often been a primary way to express oneself.[1] And for gay men, most of whom don't have children, the desire for some meaningful way to engage with the world is often an ongoing quest.

It's easy for men to identify with their profession. Our persona as a lawyer, a teacher, a scientist becomes our identity. This identification with our profession can be very satisfying, but it can also create a crisis when it's no longer fulfilling or when outward circumstances, such as layoffs, disability, or changes in the economy make it impossible to continue.[2]

At midlife we're often at the peak of our careers. We may have a lot of satisfying accomplishments, material goods, and financial stability. Yet some men begin to wonder, "Is this all there is?" For many men at midlife, work begins to recede in importance in their overall sense of well-being.[3] Some men find that their interests shift to relationships and friends or to volunteer work, or they develop a more spiritual sense of meaning in their lives.

The following examples show a range of shifting attitudes toward work: Steve talks about how he was more idealistic when he was younger, whereas at midlife he's becoming more practical and realistic about his accomplishments. Victor feels that he's in a place now where he can define for himself what's ethical or what isn't in his profession.

Steve: There's been a shift since I first started off in medical school. At that time I wanted to heal people. At midlife I've found myself giving up more noble, youthful ideals, and becoming more practical.

In medical school we made fun of the "LMD"—local medical doctor—who went to medical school 20 years ago and is no longer really up on the latest treatments. Now I realize I'm an "LMD." This is humbling. I can see younger people who are doing better stuff, and I'm able to appreciate their rising stars without feeling jealous.

I don't need to read and know everything. The number of professional journals I subscribe to has gone down, and I throw out journals and magazines instead of saving them. I choose certain areas where I do keep up, but for the rest, I just read the abstracts. I don't read books anymore; I read book reviews.

My research has been good, but it hasn't been picked up by the major media, while others do trashy studies and get lots of attention. I feel some resentment, but I'm not bitter. I've constructed some good foundations that will last for a while, which others can build on.

Victor: At midlife I've created the structures I needed—a profession with all the right credentials, so I can convince anyone that I can do whatever I want. Now I get to deconstruct all these structures. I have my own sense of what's ethical, and I look carefully at professional constraints to see whether I can live with them. I can run off to Bali, do age-inappropriate things like dancing all night, even challenge the assumed wisdom of the authorities in my profession.

Randy: I'm wiser than I was when I was younger, and I can still learn because now I see the utility in learning. I'm still trying to figure out what I'm going to be when I grow up. Our major accomplishments may still be ahead of us. If I eat right, exercise, and stay involved, I can have 20 or 30 very active years left. Not just golden years or playing golf at Leisure World. We're looking forward to second careers, new skills, relationships, or a new profession.

Antoine: There are possibilities, still, but I don't have as much time for as many. I probably only have one career left. I'm more keenly aware of my limits. I think I'll do something different in another year—help a friend with another screenplay, take a class on being a travel agent, or look for an art class in another city.

Kevin: I think for people who have not had a significant relationship, finding a way to express a passion that brings a sense of fulfillment is very important—whether that's through work or creativity or political involvement.

At this age I'm mature in my career. There's still room for growth, but that identity is a source of self-esteem for me, which I didn't have when I was younger. Having goals and a realistic game plan usually allowed me to build on what I had rather than making radical changes. I'm examining my career and possible changes. And I've begun to think about retiring—mentally preparing for older age.

At this point I'm completely open to new possibilities in all areas of my life. I chew up the scenery; that's what I live for. I have solid long-term friendships and a relationship, so I'm not looking for new possibilities in that area. But in terms of ideas, new cuisine, new experiences, the fact that I'm going to live for a while has given me a whole new sense of possibilities.

For men who have devoted themselves to more artistic pursuits, midlife can bring about a practical crisis if their level of success isn't sufficient to support them. They may feel torn between pursuing creative interests and the need to take care of themselves financially.

Mario: I've had the magical life of being an artist most of my adult life and never had to work at a regular job for any extended period of time. Instead of working the last 25 years, I've spent the time exploring and having great accomplishments. But I finally got a real job at age 42, 9 to 5. Now I have a little security.

I'm still performing, not creating as much as I used to. The work I've created is admired by my peers, which is more important to me than the public. It's not like I'm performing in front of thousands of people, but my work is acknowledged and recognized as a valuable contribution to the art form.

I was making a decent income as a performer, but I needed to get out of debt. When the opportunity arose to contract out for work, I took that position—then later I got hired on with benefits. Instead of putting myself to the side as I've done for years, I need to focus on taking care of myself.

Midlife can also bring about a realization that our work is not as fulfilling as we would like, and we may be tempted to look around to see if anything else appeals to us. Changing jobs for its own sake can be a form of "making up for lost time" if we haven't thought it through carefully, but for some men, a midlife career change can be one of the most fulfilling actions they have ever taken.

It's helpful to think through a change in work by getting in touch with what's missing, figuring out how a new career would make a difference and what it would take to pull it off. Sometimes our image of a new career is different from what it's actually like to do that kind of work day after day. So talking with others in the field we're considering switching to can help us make a more realistic assessment of what we'd have to sacrifice to make a significant change in our working lives at midlife.

The following example shows how Tony got in touch with regrets that he had not gone to medical school when he was younger. In the end he found a way to change careers that still allowed him to be involved with rearing his son.

Tony: I just changed careers. I went back to school at 41 and made the transition from a nurse to a physician's assistant. When I was 20 I had the impression that life would unfold in any number of ways. The world was wide open; I could do whatever I wanted. I was a waiter and had a nice lifestyle, but it wasn't fulfilling. I cringed at the idea of turning 50 and still being a waiter. I thought, this is not me—but if I didn't do something, it would be me. So I went back to school at 27 to become a nurse.

Then I was a nurse for ten years. I had a flexible schedule, lots of time off, and I was good at it. But I couldn't see doing this for the next 25 years, either. I battled with the idea of going to medical school in my late 30s versus becoming a physician's assistant. I finally decided against going to medical school because it was a nine-year commitment that would have made me unavailable to raise my son. I would have been poor the whole time, plus the idea of trying to start a practice when I was approaching 50 wasn't very appealing.

When I started the physician's assistant program, I was very up for it at first, but then I fell into a horrible depression. I hated it and didn't think I could do it. But I didn't indulge those negative beliefs, like you're going to do horrible, you're not going to pass, because I know myself now. I just started taking one assignment at a time and didn't let myself spiral down and get overwhelmed. I couldn't have done that ten years ago. And I'm so thrilled I finished the program I chose instead of going to med school.

◆   Mentoring   ◆

Because of the separation of age groups in our community, there are not many opportunities for mentoring younger gay men. Older gay men may fear being seen as "chicken hawks," and younger men often feel dismissed because of their lack of experience. One of the challenges facing our community is trying to establish settings in which we can appreciate the knowledge and experience of both younger and older gay men.

Being a mentor for younger people, whether they are embarking on a career or simply expressing interest in a shared hobby or avocation, can be a very satisfying way of engaging with others and expressing generativity. By offering our time, guidance, and encouragement, we provide a legacy of our expertise and achievements.

Andrew: I'd like to find a way to do that. I do it in my work. It would be nice to establish a relationship with younger guys who are just coming into the community. It's like the tradition of the elders—we don't have a lot of opportunities for that.

Victor: I have a lot of young friends. I feel accepted as an equal—not discriminated against on the basis of my age. I'm the one who's often turned to when something needs to be worked through. I get to parent in a way that I wish everyone could be—and also maintain my equal relationship. One friend who's 26—his whole life is about partying, finding sex partners, and mating, which I'm not really into anymore. Yet at the same time, I'm one of the most significant figures in his life. It's a lot of fun, and our encounters always have substance.

I know that part of the connection has to do with our age difference. The last time we got together he asked me how old I was. When I told him I was 44, he said, "My God, you're as old as my mother! I can't believe I'm hanging out with someone the same age as my mother." The fact that I can do it in the way I do it gives me a unique position in their lives. I'm both older and a chum. I get invited to parties or group dancing, and it's glorious.

Randy: When I was coming of age, we had civil rights, then the antiwar, feminist, and gay movements. Most gay men I knew were trying to do something helpful, thinking of society as a whole. It was part of the zeitgeist of the age. Nowadays it seems more difficult for young people to identify with any meaningful movements for social change.

This summer I invited six nieces and nephews for a two-week trip to open their eyes to the wider world. And to make myself clearer to them as a person, not just an uncle who brings gifts at Christmas, but a real person with his own life.

They're in their early teens, and I'll be an alternative to their parents—maybe in a lifesaving way, because I suspect at least one of my nephews is gay. He can see that here's a gay man who's doing OK and is not so strange, even according to our black middle-class values. You can be healthy and happy in the world without marrying in your 20s and having kids.

When I was with them, I tried not to sound like an elder, but something would slip out—not truth, exactly, something different from truth—perhaps a distilled experience that might be helpful to others.

Kevin: I entered midlife when I got out of grad school. I ended my last unhappy relationship and said, "I'm not a kid anymore, I'm not going to take any shit." I felt much more the master of my destiny than ever before in my life.

I have wonderful relationships with people around my own age and mentors who are older, who have guided me and mirrored me. My older gay friends who have made a successful adjustment have modeled this for me. Since I had mentors who told me about midlife, I was prepared for the changes that occurred. When I had certain illnesses or changes in my body, my friends would say "You're getting older, honey!" and laugh about it. I still have a sense of humor about these changes, and that goes a long way.

For myself, aging has been much more about gaining than having to let go. I scarcely notice the letting go, maybe because my mentors' influence made it so easy for me. Older and more experienced friends have had an immensely positive influence in shaping my life. I wouldn't be the same person if it hadn't been for them. It's amazing to think about.

In my love life I went from being the younger one who had power by being younger and attractive to being a caretaker for my lover who was dying. I went from being the center of universe as a younger man and more toward giving to the world. I feel the need to give back.

In my professional life I went from being a novice therapist to being a mentor for younger people. I began to see there were gains. You're not the one who's given attention for being young and vulnerable. You have to be bigger and generous, and there's fulfillment in that.

Being involved in supervising younger men has been gratifying. I like giving to younger people in my profession, and I enjoy their appreciation. They may not see me as attractive physically, but they find me attractive in terms of my experience and my generosity. My current persona contains a bit of the sage. I suppose we all need to feel grand in some way.

Antoine: I provide mentoring for my partner, even though he's older. I also feel more like a parent to his son and daughter than I used to. Both of them are grown now, but they're going through separations from their partners. Being there for them has been important for me.

Mario: The relationship I have with my 20-year-old niece is like being a mentor. She benefits from my wisdom, but I'm not parenting her. We have fun. I'm selective in terms of whom I mentor. I weigh it with humor and friendship and understanding. I'm learning not to tell people what they should do. I'm letting them do it on their own and supporting them. It's wonderful to see people discover things for themselves. I can be amused, not in a mocking way, but just enjoying how life works.

◆ Midlife and Beyond ◆

Midlife often brings up thoughts about retirement. Many gay men live for the moment, and it comes as something of a shock to realize that if we don't put something in place, we're going to be out in the cold. A friend of mine in his 60s once warned me, "The old you is going to be very pissed off at the young you if you don't make some sound financial plans for your retirement."

Brian: I've recently started thinking about retirement. I've never been good at this kind of planning. I'm at the halfway point of my career and want to make sure I can support myself when I retire. I'd like to write, travel, and visit friends, and be able to do things with my son.

Randy: I recently took an early retirement package after working for a company that was fairly compatible with my personal values. It's a progressive corporation that initiated compassionate treatment of people with AIDS and made it easy for gays to come out. There was a sense that you could create a respectable product and appreciate different backgrounds. Work could be creative and not soul-killing, the way most corporate life is. At the end of my year off, I'd still like to create a better marriage between what I believe in and what would earn me some money.

My severance package will allow me to take a less lucrative position once I go back to work. So I'm considering going back into teaching or something like social work. I think it's necessary for the fabric of society for us to share and try to improve things for others who are in a much more desperate situation. I've worked with young people, arts organizations, senior citizens, Project Open Hand, and I'd like to see if I can combine my corporate skills with my volunteer interests.

One of my goals during my time off is to document our family history. For a lot of African-Americans, just saying we're descended from slaves seems nebulous. Our family is partly African, Native American, and European. As black people we can relate to Adam Clayton Powell or Langston Hughes, but it becomes more cogent when it's your own great-grandfather. They don't have to be famous, but just knowing what kind of people they were—like whether they liked jazz or played the blues, whether they were religious or not. I'm the only one in my family who has the time and training to do this.

I'd originally thought, "Yippee, I have all this time to myself," but the truth is, it can feel very isolating. The rest of the world gets up and goes to work on Monday. I'm relieved, yet feel left out. Who am I now that I'm not working? I'd like to spend time on more conscious reflection—finishing poems, trying to develop some friendships to a deeper level.

Mentoring is an example of generativity, which is a way of consolidating our accomplishments and giving back to the larger community. We'll explore this in more detail in the final chapter.

Relating These Themes to Your Own Experience:

- What kind of work did you imagine you'd be doing when you were younger?
- What are you doing now?
- What else do you wish you could have tried?

- What else do you want to do now?
- What opportunities do you have in your life for mentoring younger people?

Notes

1. In his longitudinal study of male development, George Vaillant also identified "intimacy and career consolidation" as major tasks. *Adaptation to Life* by George Vaillant. Boston: Little, Brown, 1977.

2. For more about the liability of identifying with one's professional persona, see *The Archetypes and the Collective Unconscious* by Carl Jung, p. 123. Princeton: Princeton/Bollingen, 1980. Jung suggests that "the construction of a suitable persona means a formidable concession to the external world, a genuine self-sacrifice which drives the ego straight into identification with the persona, so that people really do exist who believe they are what they pretend to be." See *Persona* by Robert Hopcke, p. 16.

3. In a study of men in their 40s, researchers found that many men were satisfied with their jobs but unhappy with their lives. *Men in Their Forties* by Lois Tamir. New York: Springer, 1982.

CHAPTER 10

GAY MEN AS SHAMAN/TRICKSTERS

As young gay men we often set out on our journey with confidence and bravado, looking for worlds to conquer and dragons to slay. We tend to be single-minded, full of energy, and ready to do battle with anything that gets in our way. Once we've come out, it's our time to overthrow the patriarchy and have our day in the sun. For many younger gays, this phase is often exemplified by in-your-face activism, along with wild styles of hair, music, and dress.

At midlife we no longer need to prove ourselves with strength and derring-do. We shift from a stance of self-protection (that was necessary for our very survival as young men) to a sense of grounded self-confidence in our gay identity. We know who we are and are more self-accepting.

We have a greater perspective on which to draw, but we also become more aware of what we don't know. Part of our wisdom at midlife lies in being more humble about our assessments of life and others. Our prior confidence in the lasting truth of our opinions begins to fade. In contrast to our youthful identity, in which any feeling that contradicted our conscious self-image tended to be suppressed, there's a greater tolerance for seemingly contradictory views: We can be both masculine and feminine, loving and angry, strong and vulnerable.[1] This greater tolerance helps to counter internalized homophobia and allows for a deeper acceptance of our sexual orientation. It also allows us to be more accepting of other points of view—there are many ways to be gay.

In this chapter we'll look at how our midlife role is exemplified by the trickster, or wounded healer. Then we'll cover midlife tasks, such as generativity and the search for meaning, to round out our journey.

◆ Tricksters and Wounded Healers ◆

In his book *Beyond the Hero,* Allan Chinen describes how men at midlife can grow beyond the hero archetype by transcending patriarchal values. Rather than using strength and power to overcome our adversaries, we often resort to wit, cunning, and wisdom. The trickster provides a creative alternative to the autocrat. Instead of imposing his will, he's willing to listen, experiment, and explore.[2] He also tricks us into a new perspective and keeps us from taking ourselves too seriously.[3]

Throughout the world, folk tales demonstrate the role of the trickster as a shadow figure: a wounded healer, shaman, mentor, or source of generativity. The emphasis is on healing rather than heroism, communication rather than conquest, exploration rather than exploitation, and generativity rather than glory.[4]

These are all natural shifts at midlife—when we no longer have to prove ourselves, our influence makes itself felt more subtly—through skillful means, "crazy wisdom," and empathy.[5]

It struck me that gay men's path of development reflects the trickster/shaman archetype of traditional cultures. By healing the wounds of homophobia, discrimination, and multiple loss, gay men at midlife can also serve as wounded healers. Because the wounded healer accepts his own vulnerability, he expands his capacity for compassion. Rather than being judgmental or contemptuous toward other gay men who are still suffering from internalized homophobia, we can recognize ourselves in their internal conflicts. We can extend this sense of compassion to younger gay men who are still struggling to find their place in the world and also extend it to one another when we're groping about at midlife, trying to find our own way through the dark wood.

The gay subculture has many examples of gay men taking on the role of imp, trickster, or clown. Drag shows and camp figures such as the Angels of Light or the Sisters of Perpetual Indulgence have used humor to reflect, satirize, and poke fun at the patriarchy. Irony abounds in gay cultural products, which are often self-reflexive, winking at the audience, with humor and self-deprecation.

Drag queens subvert our "sacred" gender expectations. Drag is also a way of recognizing the anima in ourselves and others. Rather than demeaning women, drag queens frequently make fun of straight men's stereotypes of women and gay men. They also acknowledge our own shadow figures, such as the bitchy queen.

American culture tends to devalue and disown certain qualities, such as creativity, trickery, and humor. When we subvert gender roles, for example, we hold a mirror up to society by reflecting its own projections. We're seen as threatening, rather than being understood as a natural correction to a hypermasculine, patriarchal culture. Examples include the furious controversies over Robert Mapplethorpe's exhibitions, and the backlash against funding of "homosexual art" by the National Endowment for the Arts. We are scapegoated by the religious right as a danger to the family, spreaders of disease, and child molesters.[6]

We are an easy target for society's shadow projections because the patriarchy by its very nature tends to suppress unacceptable impulses in favor of the outward rules. These rigid rules tend to neglect the realities (and varieties) of human nature, creativity, and sexuality. The denied impulse is likely to reemerge through outlaws, outsiders, and tricksters, who are then seen as demons or in league with the devil.

The Daemon

In many cultures there is a "demonic" aspect to healing.[7] Psychologically, the "daemon" can be understood as an upsurge in unconscious shadow material. Through various rituals, these split-off images and impulses are reintegrated into the personality, and the person is healed. These therapeutic practices are usually led by a shaman figure, who has been initiated into curative lore following his own healing crisis.

In some forms, consensual sadomasochism can be understood as a form of "demonic" healing. Certainly, many people simply enjoy exploring the line between pleasure and pain, and not all S/M reflects a reenactment of early abuse. But some men who were abused as children may find themselves drawn to S/M as a way to master previous trauma. By taking on either role and controlling the reenactment with a trusted partner, S/M can replace early victimization with a sense of empowerment, control, and safety.

Instead of understanding its power for healing, Christianity split off the daemon and equated pagan trickster figures, witches, and shamans with the devil.[8] Similarly, in modern times sadomasochism has been pathologized. This process of demonization can be understood as a projection of the shadow. The wider culture projects its unacceptable impulses onto scapegoated groups. For example, it sees gay men as preoccupied with sex, ignoring its own sexual contradictions. When sexual impulses are split off and denied, it often results in the curious blend of Puritanism and sex obsession we see in American culture today. As exemplified by the recent "scandal" over discussing masturbation in public schools, everybody's doing it, but nobody wants to talk about it.[9]

Throughout history we can see many ways in which homosexuality has been demonized as the "other." But some cultures provide a space for the daemon to emerge: through dance, trance, and healing practices. Numerous anthropological studies confirm that in traditional cultures, the "two-spirit" person of ambiguous sexuality often filled this role of healer or shaman.[10]

Trusting Our Inner Guidance

When viewed within the context of the wider culture, part of what gay men represent is a quality of trusting one's inner daemon, will, or guidance, in contrast to outward authority, rules, and judgment. Trusting our inner guidance is a common theme at midlife.

Whenever this interior source of inspiration is recognized, it threatens the current orthodoxy. This can be seen in the conflicts between religious traditions throughout history. In Christianity, for example, the Gnostics believed in listening to one's own inner light, whereas the church set up specific dogmas, such as the Apostles' Creed, and lines of authority to conduct the sacraments. These rules defined what it meant to be a Christian, and any deviation was seen as heresy.[11]

Gay people must pay attention to our "inner light" in order to come to terms with our sexual orientation. We are a direct threat to dogma because we stand outside the authority of church doctrine, claiming our own internal guidance.[12] By the time we reach midlife, we are in a good position to let this inner light shine, illuminating the world around us with our self-confidence and well-earned wisdom.

Shaping the Culture

Patriarchal culture rejects the trickster and gay men—yet it also depends on us for art, theater, dance, fashion, and many other cultural artifacts and events. There is a curious paradox in the fact that much of our cultural life is influenced by a gay sensibility—especially when it's disguised or transmuted into terms that seem comforting or familiar. Yet some pieces are permeated with a tragic ethos, and they become icons for gay longing. In *The Wizard of Oz,* Dorothy exclaims, "We're not in Kansas anymore!" We yearn for a real home, "somewhere over the rainbow," with people who really understand us.

Many gay men at midlife have developed new rituals for celebrating our roles as shamans from various traditions. Although some people object to using elements of traditional cultures in these flights of fancy, two-spirit people have contributed to many of these traditions in the past. This playful impulse carries through the culture we are now creating. Fairy gatherings, spiritual retreats, and gay summer camps have developed rituals for representing our connections to nature, for celebrating our sexuality, for healing from homophobia, and for fighting AIDS. On a lighter note, outrageous drag, nudity, and self-mockery reveal the trickster spirit in our talent shows.

As gay men at midlife, we often feel as though there's no place for us, even within our own community. Yet midlife can be understood as a return once again to a sense of inner guidance. The archetype of the trickster shows us how to transcend the hero, who has to prove himself by overpowering his adversary. The trickster also subverts the overbearing, imperious patriarch, who establishes a dogmatic authority, demanding respect and recognition. In its place the trickster provides a model for midlife generativity, nurturing, and cunning. Our experience of midlife can provide the gay community with a natural influence in a more subtle, sometimes impish way that draws us together in mutual support, compassion, humor, and healing.

◆ Midlife Tasks ◆

As mentioned earlier, during midlife the "persona" moves toward a more authentic self—we let go of our masks and become truer to ourselves. At the same time, even though we're less dependent on outward approval, this sense of authenticity is not necessarily selfish. Because we're more in tune with what's really satisfying, authenticity leads toward generativity rather than self-aggrandizement. This shift—from outward conformity to inner vitality and authentic sharing—can be very gratifying.

To get to this sense of authentic sharing, it helps to work through some of the following tasks. And we can best approach these tasks in a context of mutual support—by reaching out to other men to talk about the changes in our lives.

Midlife tasks for gay men:
- Come to terms with regrets
- Experience humility without humiliation
- Develop generativity
- Reach out to others
- Balance engagement with detachment
- Find a sense of meaning/spirituality
- Gain authenticity and equanimity
- Leave a legacy

Come to Terms With Regrets

Among many other aspects we've explored, midlife is also a time of coming to terms with regrets—things left undone, dreams unfulfilled, and mistakes made along the way. At the same time we can recognize our own strength and wisdom, transforming the past by seeing it for what it was rather than blaming ourselves or others. We can deal with it rather than using it as an excuse for not continuing or becoming bitter.

At midlife there is often a growing equanimity and acceptance of past mistakes, with some insight that given who we were at the time, there may not have been much else we could have done differently. We can recognize the real impact of homophobia on our development and how that might have limited our perception of what was possible. And we can use our current insight to support our determination to live our lives now in the most fulfilling way.

Tony: I wish I could have carried less shame. I know you can't just say "I'm not going to be ashamed anymore" and be done with it. But I realize how my own frame of mind influences my experience at the gym or just walking into a room. I wish I could have made that shift when I was younger.

I wish I had been together enough to go to medical school in my early 20s. I would have preferred to have become a physician, so I was unable to achieve the goal I wanted. There's something kind of sad about that. I just wasn't confident enough to pursue this career earlier. When I was 20 I was just hating myself.

At this point in my life, I feel pretty comfortable with the decision not to go to medical school at 40. Instead of a big struggle, I have time to do things I enjoy—travel, getting together with friends, going to movies and plays, going to the beach. I enjoy all that, and if I had gone to med school, I would be very unhappy. So I'm glad I decided not to go, at this stage in my life.

Since I made that decision, I'm more a part of my son's life. I can participate in his day-to-day struggles and support him in ways I wish I could have been supported while I was growing up. I get a tremendous amount of fulfillment from that. If I'd gone to med school, I wouldn't have been available for him. I had to let go of one dream when I decided not to be a physician, but I'm getting back other things that are so much more important. Medicine has a hierarchy, and I'd rather be at the top, but now I'm actually doing much of the work of a medical doctor, which is very fulfilling. I see patients on my own, diagnose and treat them. The only thing missing is the social status associated with being a physician, and I guess my goal is for that not to matter.

Brian: I could have been bolder when I was younger, especially in terms of dating and expressing sexual interest, but in fact I wasn't ready to. I'd like to have started this idea of having a child earlier.

Kevin: When I graduated from college, I wish I would have gone for a Ph.D., but I wasn't ready. I wish I could have been more studious—but I wasn't. In some ways it's all been necessary—I just did what I needed to do to get by at the time, and I can wish things were different, but they weren't. I'm pretty OK with that now.

Victor: I like my life, though there are certain elements I might like better—a more stable source of income, for example—and sometimes I wonder if I should have gotten a degree in business. Yet everything I've done has created my life. If I like it now, in a way it's foolish to want to change a particular piece of it. The main point is that I feel content, and if I'd made different decisions maybe I wouldn't feel that way. It was through the decisions that I made that I reached this level of satisfaction. I feel fortunate because whatever I've done, through hard work or meditation, I've been able to reach this feeling of contentment, even though I'm not in touch with it at times.

Andrew: I wish I'd been financially more skillful—so I could be more independent and enjoy my 50s and travel. Money doesn't bring happiness, but it can bring freedom. I play it too safe—I want to take more risks.

Steve: I wish I'd been more extroverted, more sociable—but then I might be dead. I regret not having more fun, although that would have been hard to do in medical school. I wish I'd developed more close friends when I was younger, although I'm doing that now.

Randy: I wish I'd taken more risks in my 20s, joined the Peace Corps, traveled in the rural south, and interviewed civil rights leaders, as I had an offer to do. Except for not getting married, I tended to take the more familiar or safer route.

When I was in college, I was part of a small minority in a white elitist school. When students took off to bum around the country or go to Europe, I thought that was a rich, white-boy thing. They could always come home and get a job, but that didn't seem like it was a realistic option for me. I felt I had to be serious and move along with my career. Now I'm sorry I didn't take off some time and travel around.

I wish I'd had a longer relationship—the longest was a year. I'd enjoy the deepening of appreciation that can happen in a healthy relationship. When I think of the people I know who have found someone, it was luck or possibly an openness or flexibility I didn't have. It's not as though I stood around rejecting lots of possibilities. Maybe I was overlooking people who were available and idealized some men who were out of reach. I'm not sure that pattern isn't continuing.

Experience Humility Without Humiliation

Similar to the process of grief, we can experience disappointments without lowering our self-esteem. We can get in touch with our limitations without blaming ourselves. In contrast to the grandiosity and self-deprecation cycle of youth, we can experience both success and failure with equanimity: If we're successful, we're naturally glad, but we don't assume that means we're better than anyone else. And if we fail, we grieve the loss, but without assuming we're any less worthwhile as human beings. The natural disappointments in life tend to undermine the grandiosity of youth. But the sting of disenchantment is soothed at midlife by the balm of a more realistic self-acceptance. Through self-acceptance, we can acknowledge our human frailties and personal limitations, experiencing humility without feeling humiliated.

Kevin: I think midlife involves accepting some dissatisfaction. It's a way of reframing expectations philosophically. For example, a man's current work situation might not be the ideal he had in mind when he was younger, but it provides money and security.

When we're young we have a lot of experiences where our youthful ideas, illusions, and normal grandiosity get cut down to size. And that's very painful. My grandiosity has experienced a great deal of erosion over the years. I'm at the point now where there's still enough left to have fun with, but I've been forced into a position of humility in a lot of ways, and that's a gift of age. Now I know how to avoid humiliating circumstances, although it's not always with humility.

Hal: It's better than ever before—I don't feel success or failure means anything about me. That's especially shifted around my body. I used to be completely identified with my body and anything it did—if I was fat or thin, hard or soft, I felt much more vulnerable. Now, whether or not I fit some gay prototype, I feel that my body's OK just how it is.

If others attempt to shame me by identifying me with my body, that just falls flat because there's no charge for me. But if you already have doubts about yourself, that's when it feels humiliating. They've nailed you in exactly the place where you're already vulnerable.

Andrew: One of my teachers said, "Feeling embarrassment and healthy shame is a prerequisite for having a relationship with God." Without humility we're good enough on our own, which means we don't have to have a relationship with something greater. Humility takes away our grandiosity. Because I've dealt a lot with my shame, it's not something I have to hide from myself and others.

Victor: One's sense of self gets broader and healthier even in face of difficult situations. I think I have a self—this is who I am—that is the core belief that we grasp on to, and it's the cause of suffering. To the extent that life forces us to expand our sense of self, that's good.

Develop Generativity

Erik Erikson, in his studies of human development, identified generativity as the major task of midlife, following the consolidation of intimate relationships.[13] Heterosexual men often see their role as parents within the family as a major way for them to express their generativity. However, gay men usually need to consolidate a gay identity before we're able to resolve the developmental task of "isolation versus intimacy" that Erikson cites as the primary task of young adulthood. Because of the delay that many gay men experience in coming to terms with our orientation, we may still be working on establishing intimate connections at the same time we're dealing with generativity.[14]

As mentioned in the previous chapter, mentoring is one way of getting in touch with our desire to contribute something to others. Generativity is also expressed through gay men's ability to engage creatively with the surrounding society—through work, volunteering, or creative expression.

Andrew: What's my place in my community? What contribution can I make, now that I'm older? I think of things to teach that I've learned and how I can pass that on. Whenever I learn something, I always assume everyone else knows that already, and now I do too. As I talk with people, I realize that's not true. So I'm thinking more about what I've learned that would be exciting for me to teach others.

Kevin: It's a time of reevaluation—of work, a sense of meaning, self-worth, and one's place in the gay community. I knew a man who was losing his looks and got totally freaked out because it was hard to see what other values he has. I can see that now my self-esteem has less to do with physical attraction, which has been replaced by other values, like generativity. Generativity for me means giving back, volunteer work, or other modifications in my career.

Antoine: I got involved with the same-sex marriage movement here in Hawaii. We were trying to get the legislature not to have a constitutional convention, which they could use to circumvent the Hawaiian supreme court and stop the legalization of gay marriage. I was pretty focused on that until I developed this eye trouble. Getting involved with this project was a form of generativity for me. The gay youths today don't know who Liza Minnelli and Judy Garland were. They just threw themselves into work without any pretenses. I thought it was refreshing. I liked the way they think. It's something new coming up.

Randy: I felt a certain burden coming from a prominent family. I had relatives who were doctors, corporate executives; there were scholarships and schools named after my father, plus I was the oldest son. So I was supposed to be a community leader and a role model.

When my parents thought I might go into the ministry they were happy about it. Being a minister is one of the most prestigious roles you could choose in the black community. It connects to the community as well as being a spiritual path. Teaching was not quite as good but still respectable.

I see the first phase of life still living with parents, untested in what I really believed or how I'll behave. Then phase two was during my 20s and 30s—interesting work, nonprofit involvement, travel, and delights of the flesh. Now in phase three, I can more consciously select my life, my work, level of pleasure, relationships, and contributions.

Because I've been lucky in my life, I've been charitable and socially conscious, but haven't made any particular mark outside of my friends and family. I had a strong start with my family and other gifts, and I'd like to give back to the world in the proportion to what I've been given. I have this sense that if I don't do something along these lines in the next ten years, it's not going to happen.

I'd like to articulate my thoughts about the world in a way that could be shared—whether through a book or poetry or politics, I'm not sure. Teachers, like parents, make a contribution through the children we teach and influence. I still have some hope of becoming a really good teacher or describing a kind of pedagogy that will help people learn and appreciate what's important.

Hal: My whole life is about giving to others. I work in the gay community, and that's where I'm trying to have the biggest impact. I never was a part of bars or gay pride when I was younger. I never knew about the Stonewall riots until I was much older. There was nothing out there for gay men to do for themselves— it was always about the group or the community and not about themselves as individuals. What's missing is the importance of being an individual. Coming from yourself first, not being narcissistic or self-obsessed, but having self-love and self-respect. Self-reliance rather than comparing yourself with others.

Tony: I don't see my world getting smaller, as often happens with a close-knit group of friends. I see this as a time when I'm moving out of myself and into the world, rather than into myself. I look forward to more adventure, to broadening my horizons. I've traveled to the third world and worked with populations right here in San Francisco that have expanded my perspective. Through work I've interacted with drug addicts and pregnant women with HIV, children who don't have enough to eat, homeless people, and very poor members of minority groups. I'm looking forward to more of that.

The idea of getting married to another man and just playing bridge with other couples and going on ski trips and gay cruises doesn't really appeal to me. Of course I would like to get married, have friends over, even go on cruises, but I also want to develop my understanding and participate in the broader world. When I was younger, I used to think upper middle-class, gay, and homeless were all mutually exclusive, you either had to live in one world or another, and now I don't see it that way.

For some men, who have always been focused on taking care of others to the neglect of their own needs, taking care of themselves may be the most important thing they can do at midlife.

Mario: It's been reversed for me. I don't need a cause. I had my causes—sometimes I think about getting involved with something, but I'm more focused now on taking care of myself.

Reach Out to Others

Related to generativity is the importance of reaching out to others. One of the biggest complaints I hear from gay men at midlife is that they have a sense of isolation. Many of their friends have died, and they may still be grieving from the overwhelming impact of multiple losses. At the same time they may no longer feel comfortable in the most visible venues, such as bars and dance clubs. It takes effort to reach out, and that's hard to do when you're feeling demoralized. It's important to get support—through support groups, psychotherapy, or friends—so we don't feel so isolated. Regardless of whether we have a "primary relationship," friendship can add a tremendous richness to our lives. It takes a lot of effort, but it's possible to rebuild a sense of community with new friends.

Antoine: Most of my friends are better friends now than years ago. I'm part of their world, and they're a part of mine. It's nice to be able to depend on them.

Balance Engagement With Detachment

Another task is to balance our desire for engagement with a sense of detachment—not indifference, but a realistic assessment of our true abilities and likely effects. We can be totally engaged but detached from the "glory," if you will, of a specific outcome.

An aspect of this challenge is to be engaged with the world and with other people while at the same time detaching ourselves from the need to control them. We can exert some influence by clearly stating our own preferences, but ultimately we cannot control what other people do or how they perceive us. Usually by midlife we're not quite so concerned about that, anyway.

Hal: That's what I'm working on right now. I feel like I engage a little too much and need to detach a little bit more. For example, caring about someone's process or breakthrough more than they care about it themselves.

Victor: I see these as two sides of the same coin. It's not a question of balance—it's really not possible to be truly engaged unless you are detached. For example, I'm less engaged with my lover because I'm so attached. We have more glitches in our relationship than I have with any of my friends. Of course, because we're lovers, we interact on many more dimensions than I do with my friends. But when I'm too attached to a certain outcome, I just want him to be different and see things my way. Because I'm so attached to my own scenario, I'm not really engaged with him.

To be really engaged with someone, you can't be grasping. You have to be present for whatever comes up and not insist that it has to come out in a certain way. When I'm in my right mind, I can sit back for a moment and recognize that a particular issue is coming up and that's simply what we have to deal with.

Brian: I'm not doing such a good job balancing these aspects. I really don't want to be more detached. I always want to do more than I have time for. I have trouble accepting limitations—I get overextended and don't go into as much depth as I could. I know a little bit about a lot of things. I admire those who have a real focus, who have a lot of wisdom about fewer things, but it's just not my personality type.

Find a Sense of Meaning/Spirituality

Many gay men find themselves attracted later in life to spiritual pursuits or the quest for a sense of meaning—this despite the fact that most of the world's major religions tend to take a harsh view of homosexuality, if not condemning it altogether. But the desire for meaning, the yearning for transcendent experience, and the spiritual impulse seem to go beyond sectarian or dogmatic concerns.

Gay men have been very creative in our ability and willingness to adapt various forms of spiritual practices to our own use regardless of their origins. For some, this involves traditional religion, meditation practices, spiritual retreats, or integrating sex with spirituality. Others may not conceptualize meaning in terms of religious belief or spirituality. Their sense of meaning may derive from their personal ethics, friendships, work, love, creative expression, or an appreciation of nature and our place in the cosmos.

Brian: I've always been committed to finding meaning. It fits my personality. I was a philosophy major and a reflective type. Part of my integrity (and my class privilege) is that I've never worked at a job that felt meaningless. I'm grateful to have been able to lead my life this way. I can't imagine spending a life working at something I didn't believe in.

In some ways I can't take credit for these values. I came of age during the '60s, during this massive economic boom. I didn't need to worry about a job. I could explore the meaning of life, in contrast to the '50s, when our parents were so preoccupied with security that they had a very different sense of what was really important. We wanted to end violence and oppression and war. To my parents, who went through the depression and World War II, that was a naive luxury.

I see myself nowadays facilitating personal growth more than healing. Younger people often work on healing the wounds from their families, and I deal with a lot of that. But at midlife gay men are more often looking for meaning in life. I think if one has self-awareness and good luck, that the longer one lives, the closer one comes to finding one's own meaning.

Andrew: As I've gotten older I've put more emphasis on my spiritual practice—that's where the extra effort pays off. I look at what gives my life meaning: friends, meditation, and being in the moment. Everyone has to struggle with that. Without that sense, things are meaningless—and that becomes a fertile ground for bitterness and despair, for becoming withered.

The joys in the world are wonderful, but they're only a shadow of what it's like to be connected with God or the Infinite— so why not go for the source. Those are just words, yet I have some experience that has shown me there's a lot of truth in that.

Hal: Self-knowing, knowing myself spiritually, has been an asset and an anchor. This physical world is not all of it—only a piece of the whole thing. I see that I'm connected to everything. Bernie Siegel asks, "If you were to die tomorrow, what is the thing you were supposed to do here?" I ask myself this, What's my purpose. Living your truth and making sure it's consistent.

Kevin: A sense of meaning derives from my sense of ethics, which may refine over the years, but they're basically in place. It's part of knowing who you are. I don't miss having a spiritual life. But I do get a sense of meaning from loving relationships. It can be as casual as someone at work who I have feelings of love for and know that they care for me. I believe in human connection and charity and mutuality.

Antoine: Too many things are going on. I'm not looking for meaning as to why I'm alive—I'm just too busy to get through the day. If I can enjoy life, I do—if there's some way I can help, I'll do that.

Steve: I don't have to find meaning in everything anymore, like I did when I was young. Some things can just be fun— watching *Buffy the Vampire Slayer* or sci-fi movies. My own sense of meaning disappeared when I was raging against my disability. But now it's reconstituted and no longer intrapsychic. I'm interested in doing research that includes more social and cultural stuff. Of course, there's some grandiosity in making comments on society as a whole.

Mario: What's my purpose? My horoscope said I would discover my sense of purpose soon. Well, I hope so, because I don't have a clue as to what that is! My purpose has been in my relationships. Sometimes it's very clear—bail so-and-so out of jail. Or talking about life on the phone, eating popcorn. I have a disdain for religious institutions and manipulations that makes the word *spirituality* so difficult for me. I believe in a higher being, but it has a sense of humor. I think that's when my higher being kicks in—when I can laugh about it.

When I was 19 I was totally in angst. I climbed to the top of this mountain—it took me all day—and I sat there with my Bible and said, "God, teach me something, show me a sign." I opened the Bible and put my finger on a verse. It said, "Seek me on the mountaintop, but you will not find me." That was great. And I remember laughing and throwing the Bible in the air, and was relieved of that burden.

Gain Authenticity and Equanimity

Authenticity is one of the greatest gifts of midlife. As illustrated by the following comments, just being yourself allows for a moment-to-moment awareness. Instead of being taken out of the moment by anticipating others' judgments, authenticity enables us to act from a more centered place of self-respect, equanimity, and wisdom.

Andrew: Midlife is like being at a plateau—you don't have to run so much. You can slow down and look around. It's hard to get out of the running mode—the industriousness—which is my tendency. Working on being in the moment is as much about my own character stuff as it is about midlife.

My meditation teaching is that everything is impermanent: Everything changes, nothing lasts. But our internal experience of Being, of the Infinite, can be continuous and ever-present. That's my quest—to be more in touch with that experience in a moment-to-moment awareness.

My sense of meaning is not just about insight or values; it's experiential—a sense of peace, fullness, love, and infinity. It's vast and awesome and scary—some would call that God. It's pretty rich.

Taking things seriously and being responsible but also realizing that nothing's that important. To be able to hold both attitudes—that's been an enigma in my life, but I'm embracing it more. There's no where to go, it's all right here—I keep coming back to this.

Victor: If you insist on holding on to old structures, you'll be miserable. I believe this is true about life in general, but it's especially pertinent at midlife. Instead of propping up the corpse, realize it's heavy and it stinks, so bury it and move on.

Demanding that things stay the same, that your identity be coherent, that you always know where you're going, or that it all make sense—insisting on all that is a losing proposition. Jack Kornfield tells this story:

The Thai monk Ajarn Cha was once asked, "What does it mean not to grasp?"

He held up a crystal glass. "This is a very beautiful glass with fine handiwork. Every day I appreciate this glass. Drinking water from this glass is a special experience, because it's so fine and delicate. Yet when I look at this glass, I see it with the eyes of Buddha. Even though I return it safely to the shelf, I know it will someday break and shatter into a thousand shards. I can only really appreciate this glass if I can see it as already broken."

At this stage of my development, my previous identities are gone. I realize the way I'm talking to you today is influenced by the course I'm preparing in Buddhist psychology. One of the things about midlife is that I can better appreciate that this is not who I am; it's just me right this second. If I talked to you a few weeks ago, it would have been totally different yet just as true. When I'm in my right mind, it feels so freeing. I don't have to stand by any of this.

Leave a Legacy

A final task at midlife is often referred to as leaving a legacy. It can be wonderful to have accomplished something that has lasting influence. The trouble with the concept of "legacy" is that it lends itself to grandiose expectations about what our legacy should consist of. So it's helpful to think of "leaving a legacy" not only through great accomplishments, but simply as a reflection of the way we've lived our lives. For gay men, especially, I believe our legacy for the future is best reflected in the quality of our lives and our relationships—or to quote the Flirtations, "the love you leave behind when you're gone."

Victor: As I feel the press of time, I feel more clearly that I want to have made a contribution—something of me that persists through time. Now I've been increasingly aware that I don't have to "do" anything—every moment of my life is impacting the world around me. My young lover has been enormously affected by me—and he will continue to live his life in part because we were so intimately involved.

Andrew: I'm realizing the limits of what I can contribute to the world. I just do my little share, and it affects some people. What is it really? Just a little mark. I haven't made some huge contribution and become famous—part of me would like that, but it's not a huge regret.

Randy: People say this time of life is more realistic, but I think we should hold on to our ideals. If we can be honest and sensitive and compassionate—not necessarily as role models, but letting people see us as happy and concerned and involved—that's probably the best thing we can do, both for ourselves and for gay men in their 20s.

We should take some pride in the fact that we have created a whole new realm of possibilities for ourselves and those who come after us. They will be able to see that there are other ways of being, not some stereotype of older gays. Then maybe they'll realize, hey, these guys are being themselves, they're actively engaged and happy with the choices they've made in their lives. That makes midlife seem pretty attractive. This can be our legacy for the future.

◆ Celebrating Gay Midlife ◆

Our journey at midlife often begins with disillusionment, physical changes, and the awareness of our own mortality, which leads to the collapse of our identity as young gay men. We can try to evade our fate and hold on to our youthful persona by running amok and, when that fails, by becoming bitter. Or we can forge a new identity by grappling with our anima/animus—those neglected feminine and masculine aspects of ourselves that can round out our personality and restore a sense of wholeness: We can be more sensitive and caring toward others as well as asserting our own needs.

In the course of this passage, we also get in touch with regrets, losses, and missed opportunities. Grieving for these losses allows new growth. During this transition we can also heal our shadow side by reclaiming our projections—instead of just seeing faults in others, we can acknowledge our own deficiencies. Self-acceptance allows us to counter homophobic messages and assert our natural authority. At the same time awareness of our imperfections helps us experience humility without feeling humiliated.

Along the way, the "trickster" aspect of our crazy wisdom arrives, infusing our voyage with perspective and humor. This wisdom allows us to develop confidence in our true selves. An authentic self is the basis for evolving our own sense of generativity—finding our rightful place at midlife by giving back to the community through our insights, knowledge, creativity, and mentoring of younger men.

As gay men we bring a lot of strengths and wisdom to this transition. For many of us, midlife brings a sense of rebirth, especially after working through the various tasks we confront during this period. Ultimately, each of us has to struggle on his own to create meaning in the wilderness—and yet we can also reach out to one another. As we move along this path, we can point out potential pitfalls, share insights along the way, and leave signposts for those who follow our footsteps on this journey through the middle of our lives.

Relating These Themes to Your Own Experience:

- How do you see yourself as a "wounded healer"?
- How does your "inner trickster" serve you, in terms of humor, wisdom, or healing?
- What have been some of your regrets?

- What are you looking forward to?
- What opportunities for generativity do you see in your job and with your friends, relatives, or community?
- What are some of the sources of your own meaning in life?
- What insights and wisdom would you like to offer younger men?
- What legacy would you like to leave for the future?

Notes

1. *Beyond the Hero* by Allan Chinen, p. 89.
2. Ibid.
3. A humorous example comes from the Hopi sacred clown tradition, in which clowns wearing irreverent masks leap into a funeral or other sacred gathering. They taunt the participants with vulgar insults and poke fun at the seriousness of the event to acknowledge the shadow side and help participants keep perspective. *Beyond the Hero,* p. 72.
4. Ibid., p. 96 and 206.
5. See *Crazy Wisdom* by Wes Nisker. Berkeley: Ten Speed, Press, 1990.
6. The California State Republican Party recently adopted a resolution that opposed granting "protected minority status to persons because of their sexual orientation," and defined sexual orientation as including "practices associated with incest, sexual child abuse, bestiality, gays, lesbians, transsexuals, pedophiles, and cross-dressers among others." Cited in *San Francisco Bay Times,* March 5, 1998, p. 10.
7. *Once Upon a Midlife,* by Allan Chinen, p. 181.
8. Ibid.

9. This strange prohibition of acknowledging perfectly natural urges and practices led to the resignation of Joycelyn Elders as surgeon general after suggesting that "perhaps" masturbation should be considered as a topic of discussion in sex education and HIV prevention programs in our schools.

10. In his appeal to the United Religions Initiative to include sexual orientation, Christian de la Huerta provided a summary on two-spirit people from various cultures: "We were the shamans, the healers, the visionaries, the mediators, the peace keepers, the 'people who walk between the worlds,' the keepers of beauty. The *berdache* or two-spirit people of the Native American tribes—the *wintke* of the Lakota, the *nadle* of the Navaho, the *minquga* of the Omaha, the *hwame* of the Mohave—as well as the *isangoma* of the Zulu and the 'gatekeepers' of the Dagora in Africa, the *hijiras* in India, the *galli* priests of the goddess Cybelle...and many others were honored, respected, and even revered for the spiritual roles they fulfilled." Stanford, June, 1997. See *Coming Out Spiritually,* by Christian de la Huerta. Tarcher/Putnam, 1999. For a perspective on Native American "two-spirit" people, see *The Zuni Man-Woman* by Will Roscoe. Albuquerque: University of New Mexico Press, 1991. For a gay perspective on mythology, see *Queer Spirits: A Gay Men's Myth Book* by Will Roscoe. Boston: Beacon Press, 1995. Also, *The Mythology of Transgression: Homosexuality as Metaphor* by Jamake Highwater. Oxford: Oxford University Press, 1997.

11. The *Gnostic Gospels,* by Elaine Pagels. New York: Vintage, 1989.

12. Of course, gay men are not unique in this respect—certainly there have been many religious movements, such as the Society of Friends, that have claimed guidance by one's inner

light—and they have also been persecuted for it!

13. "Generativity is primarily the interest in establishing and guiding the next generation, although there are people who, from misfortune or because of special and genuine gifts in other directions, do not apply this drive to offspring but to other forms of altruistic concern and of creativity..." *Identity and the Life Cycle* by Erik Erikson, p. 103. New York: W.W. Norton, 1980.

14. "Given the unique issue of homosexual identity formation, such as the frequently delayed consolidation of sexual identity, the sequence of developmental tasks for a large number of lesbian and gay adults may differ from that of heterosexual adults. Some gay men...have resolved issues of generativity more fully than those of intimacy." From "Midlife Gay Men and Lesbians" by Robert Kertzner in *Textbook of Homosexuality and Mental Health,* edited by Robert Cabaj and Terry Stein, p. 293. Washington, D.C.: American Psychiatric Press, 1996.

APPENDIX

In the course of working on this project, I interviewed ten men, ranging in age from 37 to 50, to get their perspectives on the midlife transition. Of course, many gay men become acutely aware of the passing of time in their 30s and approach 40 with considerable anxiety. I've also spoken with a number of men who really felt the full force of midlife in their 50s. Although this book emphasizes the transition time of the 40s, I suspect that many gay men from their 30s to 60s will identify with these issues.

Kevin: Kevin is 41 and Irish-American. He loves music and cooking. He's a long-term survivor of HIV and has a partner of many years. They don't live together, and he prefers it that way.

Brian: Brian is 50, from an Anglo-Scottish background. He just fathered a child. He has worked for the Peace Corps, as an alternative school teacher, and as a psychotherapist.

Randy: Randy is 50 and African-American. He worked for 17 years for a large corporation and recently took a severance package to explore, travel, and figure out what he'd like to do when he gets back.

Steve: Steve is 44 and Asian-American. He works as a medical researcher.

Tony: Tony is 43 and Sicilian-American. He had a lover of 14 years who died of AIDS four years ago. At 41 he went back to school to become a physician's assistant. He coparents his nine-year old son with a lesbian couple.

Hal: Hal is 37, from a German and Irish background. He has worked as a chef and a carpenter, and now runs a personal growth seminar.

Antoine: Antoine is 45 and Hawaiian-Filipino. He works as an accountant and recently got involved with the same-sex marriage movement in Hawaii. His lover is 19 years older, and they've been together for 23 years.

Andrew: Andrew is 48 and Anglo-American. He's a body worker who teaches Yoga and meditation.

Mario: Mario is 42 and Latino. He's a dancer and choreographer who also works as a shipping clerk. His lover of ten years died three years ago.

Victor: Victor is 44 and Portuguese-American. He teaches a class on Buddhist psychology. He has a lover from Southeast Asia who is 16 years younger, and he shares his home with a longtime companion of 26 years.

Any last words, guys?

Steve: How to know you've arrived at midlife:

People call you "Sir."

Everyone under 30 looks cute.

Cops and service people look like kids.

Contemporary music seems alien.

You go into a room to get something and forget what it was.

You forget what you wanted to say.

Mountains are higher, the trails longer.

Time goes by faster.

Brian: The biggest challenge in growing older is to stay curious about what's going on rather than simply judging it. Maybe I don't like some of the changes that are happening, but I can also see that these differences have meaning.

Mario: Love thyself. To thine own self be true. Happiness starts from within. Blah, blah, blah. If you have low self-esteem or feel depressed, get help. Don't try to intellectualize it.

Tony: You don't have to stagnate—look outward, see what else is there. You can still be part of the wider world.

Kevin: Finding something meaningful is more important at this stage of life. Also, don't just be a mentor for younger men—find an older person to hang out with who's the sort of older person you want to be.

Antoine: Welcome midlife—it's not such a bad thing—growing older is just part of being alive. Live, have fun.

Victor: Be kind to yourself, compassionate with yourself. This in-between time is about the big changes that are happening in your body, in your mind, and in the unconscious parts of you that are just beginning to emerge.

Randy: I think people need to value their health. Being around seniors, you can't overestimate the value of energy and a pain-free life. If everything else is in place but you wake up in pain every day, you miss out on so much. Just take care of yourself, so you have enough energy to enjoy life.

Hal: Don't be an old geezer when you still have half your life ahead of you. You can be a geezer when you're 90. Reinvent your childhood—go skydiving, waterskiing, ballooning; play with squirt guns—all the things you wanted to do as a kid.

Andrew: Joseph Campbell said "Follow your bliss." What makes me happy is when I follow what my heart wants to do. I often do the thing that's more rational or practical, but what I'd really like to do is just go for it.